Exercise, Rest and Relaxation

Richard T. Mackey
Miami University, Oxford, Ohio

WM. C. BROWN COMPANY PUBLISHERS
Dubuque, Iowa

CONTEMPORARY TOPICS IN HEALTH SCIENCE SERIES

Consulting Editor
 ROBERT KAPLAN
 Ohio State University

Exercise, Rest and Relaxation—*Richard T. Mackey, Miami University*

Alcohol: Use, Nonuse and Abuse—*Charles R. Carroll, Ball State University*

Non-Communicable Diseases—*Wesley P. Cushman, Ohio State University*

Drugs—*Robert Kaplan, Ohio State University*

Safety and First Aid—*William T. Brennan and Donald J. Ludwig, Indiana Univeristy*

Smoking—*John T. Fodor and Lennin H. Glass, San Fernando Valley State College*

Mental Health—*James C. Pearson*

Consumer Health—*Miriam L. Tuck, The City University of New York*

Copyright © 1970 by
Wm. C. Brown Company Publishers

Library of Congress Catalog Card Number 70-110598

SBN 697–07329–7

All rights reserved. No part of this book may be reproduced in any form or by any process without permission in writing from the copyright owner.

Printed in the United States of America

Foreword

Health education is more than the primary phase of preventive medicine. Beyond the prevention of disease and the amelioration of health problems is its positive design to raise levels of well-being and liberate man's potential. Directly and indirectly it enables the individual to function most productively, creatively, and humanely.

One needs health to become educated and one needs education to develop and maintain health. Nor can one make full use of his education without it. Health is vital to the attainment of goals but we cannot preoccupy ourselves seeking it or in our obsession we shall fail to integrate all aspects of our development and performance. Health is a means to ends—the ends valued by the individual and society. Favorable modifications of health behaviors are essential to the attainment of these ends.

Contemporary Topics in Health Science offers a new and individualized format. Students and instructors can select and utilize those topics most relevant or most pertinent for the time available. Independent and class study, separately or concurrently, are enhanced by their organization. In this form they also provide greater opportunity to correlate health with other subjects.

Each book offers an up-to-date realistic discussion of currently significant health topics. Each explores its area in somewhat greater depth, with less trivia, than found in many textbook chapters. But they are designed to do more than merely present information. Within each are to be found more than partial explanations of facts. They are written by authors ranked by his professional peers as an authority in his field. They encourage the exploration of ideas, development of concepts, identifying value judgements, and selecting from a range of alternatives to enhance critical decision-making.

ROBERT KAPLAN

This book is dedicated to my father-in-law, Fred E. Oyer, whose encouragement has been a constant source of inspiration.

Contents

CHAPTER		PAGE
1	Introduction	1
2	Some Basic Understandings About Exercise	7
3	Exercise and Physical Fitness	18
4	Selecting Exercises for Your Needs	23
5	Consumer Information About Exercise Equipment	30
6	Exercise and Special Health Problems	36
7	Rest or Sleep	45
8	Relaxation	49
	Index	55

CHAPTER 1

Introduction

As a college man or woman what kind of exercise do you engage in? Perhaps you're like the man who said, "When I feel the urge for exercise I lie down until the urge passes." Why do you exercise anyway? When you're not exercising how much rest do you need? What contribution can Yoga make to your efficiency as a person? What is scientific relaxation? As you read the subsequent pages of this book, the answers to these and other questions will be forthcoming.

But first let's appraise the status of exercise habits or patterns among American college men and women today.

Exercise and College Men

If you observe men on college campuses what will you find them doing of their own volition? Team sports such as touch football, basketball and softball rank high as forms of activity. These are on an organized basis in intramural leagues and in pickup games. The closest plot of ground for touch football or softball and the handiest bankboard for basketball are used. Behind many a fraternity house and near dorms, basketball is played on makeshift courts throughout most of the academic year. Spring and fall find the tennis and golf enthusiasts in action. Some students engage in swimming during the school year, but most prefer this activity and related aquatics during the summer months.

Where courts are available, handball is a sport of great interest. Coming on very strong in recent years are Judo, Karate (Figure 4) and weight training. In the fall of 1968, the 300 men enrolled in Karate courses at Miami University were but a fraction of those enrolled in similar classes elsewhere in the nation.

College men, of course, engage in a wide variety of sports activities as part of required physical education courses. Cycling, sailing, badminton and wrestling are included in the long list. The experiences gained in these courses help to determine future participation patterns.

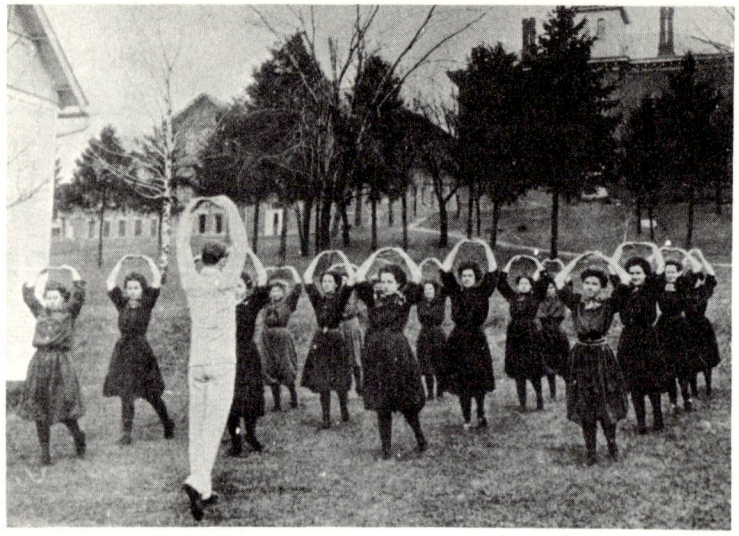

Figure 1

THEN AND . . .

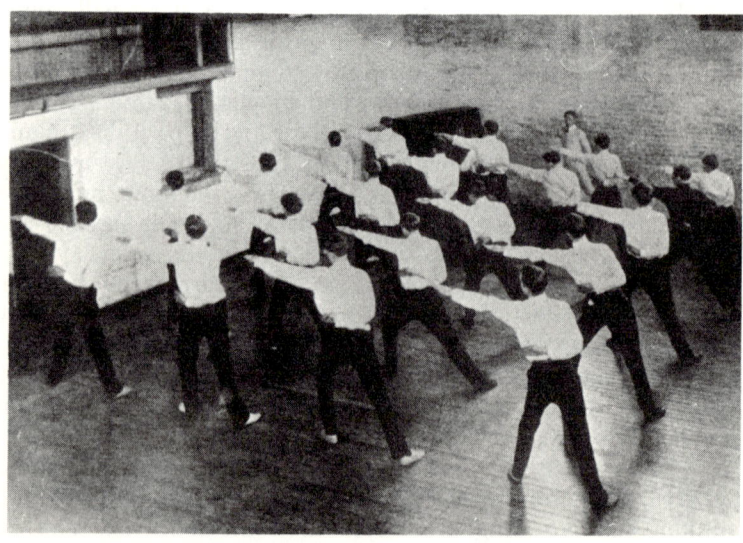

Figure 2

INTRODUCTION

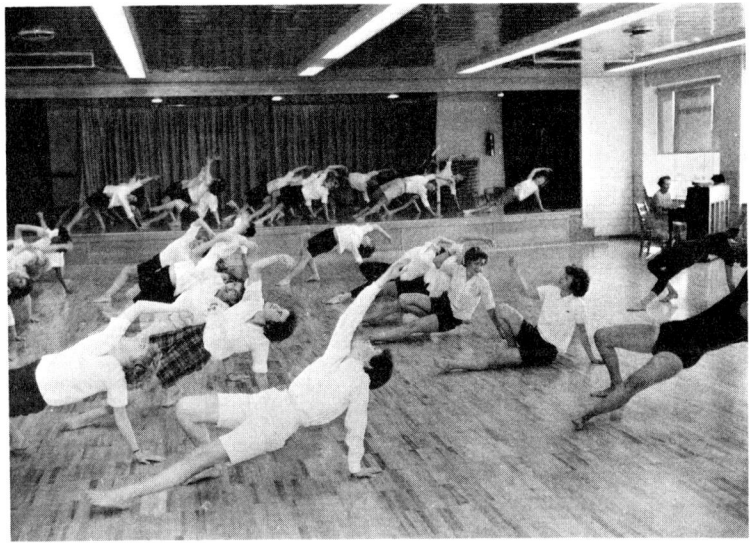

Figure 3

NOW

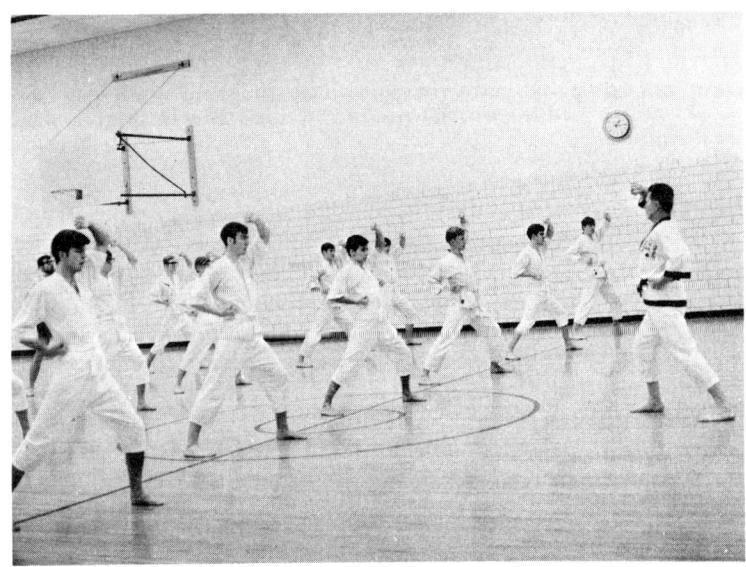

Figure 4

Exercises and College Women

When given an opportunity to select exercise-related activities, college women show some rather definite preferences. As a recreational activity, swimming ranks close to the top. Unlike the men who participate a great deal in impromptu games, women seem to prefer more organized sports. Through the Women's Recreation Association and sports clubs, college women enjoy aquatics, volleyball, bowling and dancing (Figure 3). Instructional classes which are popular include gymnastics, golf and tennis. In some colleges physical education courses in physical fitness, fundamental movement or body mechanics are receiving increased interest. Judo, Karate and Yoga also appeal to women.

Why Exercise?

As you read the foregoing pages you may have thought about your own sports participation. But have you ever analyzed why you engage in these activities? You may say, "I play tennis or swim for the exercise." If asked why you exercise, you may answer, "Because it's good for me." Are these the real reasons why you exercise? A careful probing into your motivation for participation would reveal the basic reason is ENJOYMENT. No college student or anyone else would swim, play volleyball or engage in any number of activities unless the experience was generally pleasurable. If they were doing it just for the exercise, they wouldn't continue very long.

As will be discussed later, there is much to be gained from exercise, but many of the benefits come as by-products of enjoyable or satisfying activities. Exercise is not an end in itself. Fun, enjoyment, pleasure, companionship and competition should be the prime reasons for exercise. Your goal is to improve the quality of your life through participation.

History of Exercise

If we examine man's involvement in exercise historically, we find four basic reasons for such activity. They are: (1) health, (2) military preparedness, (3) enjoyment or social values and (4) physical development.

Health. The ancient Greeks were perhaps the foremost advocates of health through exercise. In fact, Galen, a Greek born in A.D. 130, wrote a treatise "Preservation of Health and Exercise with the Small Ball," which was to influence exercise enthusiasts for centuries. The idea that through exercise people can recover from ills and weaknesses was promoted by Galen.

In more recent times, England and Scotland have promoted the health concept. The late 1800's saw the British advancing the idea that good health consists of a blending of exercise, sound nutrition and general hygiene.

American thinking in this direction was influenced by Catherine Beecher who wrote a book in 1856 entitled, "Physiology and Calisthenics for Schools and Families." Her purpose was to eliminate physical defects through formal exercise.

Military Preparedness. While the Greeks were interested in the health benefits of exercise, fitness for military purposes was also their prime concern. Socrates is reported to have said, "No citizen had a right to be an amateur in the matter of physical training; it is part of his profession as a citizen to keep himself in good condition, ready to serve his state at a moment's notice."

It is noteworthy that in American history, physical fitness related to the military has been our great concern during three major conflicts. Draft rejections because of physical defects were over 40 per cent for the Civil War, World War I and World War II. Uncorrected defects might well be associated with low physical fitness. In each case, physical training programs for service personnel and civilians were quickly initiated. During World War II, both women and men became involved in fitness programs.

Enjoyment and Social Values. Play is basic to man's nature so the recreative and social values associated with exercise have been a part of all cultures since the beginning of time. In our own culture, this aspect of exercise gains and loses emphasis as we trace our country's development. In colonial America the monotony of daily labor was eased by sports activities geared to the life of the day. These included jumping contests, foot races, rough-and-tumble fighting and wrestling matches.

The formal approach to physical training through Swedish and German gymnastics programs in the U. S. in the middle and late 1800's was followed by renewed promotion of the social outcomes of physical activity. It is interesting that the formalized calisthenics approach to exercise failed to gain the support of the masses (Figure 2). The fun of participation has continued to be important to Americans from that time to the present.

Physical Development. The Greeks were intrigued with the beauty and symmetry of the human body. Do you begin to get the idea that the Greeks had a broad outlook in the role of exercise in their society? It's true as perhaps in no other society in recorded history. As the Greeks saw it, there must be balance and harmony in the intellectual and physical aspects of man's life. When man becomes enamoured with his own body or impressed by his own intellect, he loses effectiveness as a person.

The professional strong men, the carnival buffoons and rowdies and the body-beautiful devotees who admired their own biceps are examples of over-emphasis on the physical. This narcissistic view was in evidence

Introduction

1. Why do you think there has been a surge of interest in Judo and Karate? In what sectors of your student population is the interest highest?
2. Do you think women seem to enjoy more organized sports than the impromptu variety favored by men? Why?
3. What did The Duke of Wellington mean when he said "The battle of Waterloo was won on the playing fields of Eton."
4. Why are contemporary Americans more exercise conscious than their late 19th century forefathers?

in our country among weight lifters during the middle and late 1800's and persisted until the early part of the twentieth century. The muscle men of the past have largely disappeared. The weight lifters, professional football players and shot putters of today use body development as a means of improving performance, not just for self-admiration.

Through the years, women have been more concerned with grace of movement (Figure 1), beauty of the form and flexibility than muscle size. In fact, many women have shied away from vigorous exercise because of the possibility of the development of bulging muscles. Young women like Judith Anne Ford, Miss America of 1968, who is beautiful and a beautifully formed gymnast, is proof that this fear is unfounded.

Selected Readings

HACKENSMITH, CHARLES W. *History of Physical Education.* New York: Harper and Row. 1966.

LENTZ, JOHN J. "To Exercise or Not to Exercise." *Today's Health.* March, 1963. p. 28.

CHAPTER 2

Some Basic Understandings About Exercise

If you are to make some intelligent decisions about exercise, there are facts you need to know about muscles. First, muscle tissue is elastic. Because of this elasticity, the normal resting length of your muscles can be changed through exercise. Exercises designed to shorten your abdominal muscles, for example, enable you to maintain a flat, trim waistline. The ability to stretch your muscles gives you the flexibility to perform well in activities like gymnastics and dance. Flexibility is essential to all graceful movement.

Second, muscles respond to either voluntary or involuntary nerve impulses. Involuntary muscle contraction is known as *tonus*. This state of partial contraction enables you to maintain your posture without conscious thought. Tonus, a low state of tension in your muscles, also enables you to respond quickly to a call for action. Regular exercise improves the tonus or tone in your muscles.

Third, when you contract your muscles voluntarily, usually they get shorter and thicker (Figure 5). Observe your biceps when you flex your arm. Sometimes, however, muscles lengthen as they contract (Figure 6). This happens when you bend forward at the waist from an erect standing position. After the initial shortening contraction of your abdominals to move your upper body forward, gravity takes over and your back muscles are involved in lengthening contraction.

Fourth, muscle tissue like most portions of the human organism is constantly changing. Muscles are either getting stronger or weaker. Rarely are they in a static state for very long. If you use your muscles less than usual, they will begin to *atrophy* or waste away. Some of your muscular power will be lost. This may be an almost unnoticeable change as during periods of slightly lessened activity, or quite marked if you immobilize a limb in a cast for six weeks or so because of a fracture or other injury. If your period of total body inactivity lasts for a considerable length of time, such as months or years, then, of course, the slight change becomes accumulative. For many college men and women this period of lessened activity begins during their junior and senior years.

8   SOME BASIC UNDERSTANDINGS ABOUT EXERCISE

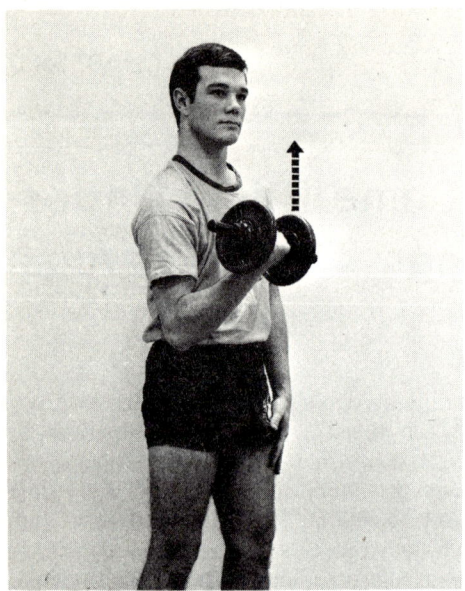

Figure 5. Shortening Contraction

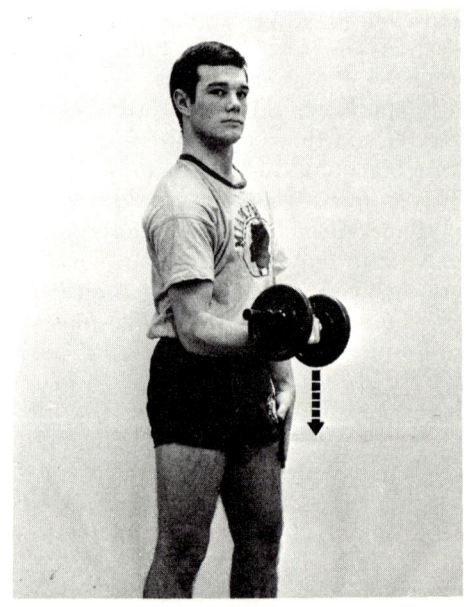

Figure 6. Lengthening Contraction

SOME BASIC UNDERSTANDINGS ABOUT EXERCISE

Fifth, a principle you must grasp is that muscles only reach higher levels of efficiency when they are "overloaded" or subjected to stress beyond the normal demands of daily living. Just how you can employ the "overload" principle will be discussed in the pages to follow.

Strength and Endurance

What is strength? What is endurance? How are they related?

Strength. Strength is defined as: the amount of force which can be applied by a muscle or, muscle group in a single maximum contraction. For example: if you stood with your arms at your side, grasped a weight such as a dumbell in your right hand and flexed your arm bringing the weight toward your shoulder, the amount of weight you can lift, *one time*, is a measure of your strength.

Endurance. Endurance is defined as: the ability to contract or use your muscles repeatedly. In our example above, the number of times that you can lift the dumbbell would determine your endurance. Actually, there are two types of endurance, *local endurance* and *general endurance*. Local endurance relates to your muscles only, while general endurance involves your muscles and your cardiovascular (heart, veins, and arteries) and respiratory systems. If you flex your index finger many times, your finger muscles will eventually become fatigued, but you won't become breathless nor will your heart pound. This is an example of *local endurance*. If, however, you hop up and down on one leg several times, not only will your leg muscles become fatigued but you'll get winded and your heart rate will speed up markedly. Your *general endurance* is shown in our second example and you can see that the difference in the two types is a matter of extent of total body involvement.

While definitions of *strength* and *endurance* indicate they are quite different, it is also true that they are interrelated. Almost any vigorous activity you engage in requires both strength and endurance. It is an interesting phenomenon that inactivity usually affects endurance much more so than strength. Even aged men and women retain rather high levels of grip strength but have very little endurance. General body exercise very quickly brings on fatigue for most aged persons.

Cardiovascular and Respiratory Changes

During generalized activity or exercise which lasts more than 30 seconds, your cardiovascular and respiratory systems must make an adjustment. Recall our example of hopping up and down on one foot. This is a vigorous activity because you are lifting your entire body weight each time you hop. After just a few hops, your body cannot carry on without increased oxygen and blood supply to the muscle cells. So your pulse rate and breathing rate speed up to meet these demands. Unlike a gasoline engine, however, which stops when the fuel is gone, your body can go into debt for oxygen when the demand exceeds the rate at which it can be supplied. This accounts for the ability of a trained individual to run 100 yards on a breath or two or to swim 50 yards under the same circumstances. In a vigorous, all-out activity of this type, your body goes into oxygen debt almost immediately and you become exhausted in a few seconds. With more moderate exercise of longer duration, your body reacts differently.

You've probably experienced this reaction of your body to extended exercise, but didn't understand just what was happening. In swimming about a quarter mile or running a mile, your body's adaptation is easily recognized. As you start to run or swim you feel fresh and full of energy. Your body makes an initial adjustment to the increased level of activity and you feel fine for a time. Then you begin to feel so tired you don't think you can continue. Your body is falling behind in reacting to the stress of activity. If you continue, however, a sort of free wheeling sensation will develop and you'll feel fine again. This is known as the second-wind phenomenon and is evidence that your body has reached a point of equilibrium between supply and demand for oxygen. If your body is not well-conditioned your second wind will not last very long. Regardless of your conditioning level, however, continued activity will eventually result in fatigue again being present. For a time after you cease running or swimming you will feel hot and your face will be flushed as your body rids itself of accumulated waste products. This is a chemical process and is another amazing mechanism of your body—the ability to recover quickly after vigorous exercise.

Types of Exercise

The important thing to remember regarding the different types of exercise presented here are the underlying principles. By understanding the principles you are better equipped to select exercises in tune with your needs.

Isometrics. Despite all the furor about isometrics in recent years, it is not really a new exercise concept. *Isometrics* may be defined as muscle contraction against resistance in which little or no movement of body parts occur. If you stand in a doorway with your hands against the door frame and push hard, you are performing an isometric exercise (Figure 7). An active child pushes and pulls immovable objects many times a day in ordinary play. This accounts in part, at least, for the differences in the musculature of children. The inactive or lethargic child doesn't use isometrics very much. A look at your fellow students will convince you that this drive for activity, or lack of it, carries on into adulthood.

The research done in Germany by Hettinger and Muller in 1953 brought isometrics into public view. According to their findings, if you exert at least two-thirds of maximum force in a single contraction once a day and hold that contraction for 6 seconds you build strength. Refer back to our definition of strength as you consider these facts.

More recent research indicates that perhaps multiple contractions of six seconds up to 5 or 10 times per day and increasing resistance from two-thirds maximum to maximum will develop higher levels of strength than with the original formula.

Unquestionably, isometrics are an efficient method of building strength. They take little time, almost no equipment and you don't need another person to assist you. They are not, however, a panacea for all of your exercise needs as many athletic coaches have discovered. *Isometrics do not contribute much to general endurance.* Some local endurance is developed; just how much no one knows at this point. If you wish to engage in sports in which prolonged exertion is necessary, isometrics aren't of much value. The place of isometrics in your exercise program will be discussed in Chapter 4.

Isotonics. Isotonics involve contraction in which movement of body parts takes place. Moving a dumbbell from your side to your shoulder by flexing your elbow is an isotonic exercise. In this case, the resistance or weight is not sufficient to prevent movement as in an isometric exercise. In both kinds of exercise the muscle is "overloaded" or is put under stress beyond normal usage. Strength is gained through isotonics.

By repeating the exercise several times, endurance is also improved. By varying the amount of resistance or weight and the number of repetitions, isotonics can be used for strength improvement or cause gains in endurance (Figure 8). The basic principle is: *For strength use high resistance and low repetitions and for endurance use low resistance and high repetitions.* Properly contrived isotonic exercises can also improve and maintain your flexibility by putting your limbs through a complete range of movement. Isometrics do not improve your flexibility. Isotonics, however, require more equipment and more time than isometrics.

Aerobics. Aerobics (with oxygen) is the newest term in exercise (Figures 9 and 10). Although the term is new, the exercises which involve aerobics have been around a long time. Men and women were doing aerobics when the first prehistoric beast gave man a long chase. If the chase was at a moderate pace and lasted several minutes, our caveman or cavewomen was making use of the aerobic principle. In discussing aerobics credit must be given to Dr. Kenneth H. Cooper, a physician and Major in the U. S. Air Force Medical Corps. Dr. Cooper's book, *Aerobics,* presents the underlying concepts backed by much research. It is a very readable book and includes extensive and easy-to-follow exercise patterns (Tables 1 and 2).

12　　　　　　　　　　SOME BASIC UNDERSTANDINGS ABOUT EXERCISE

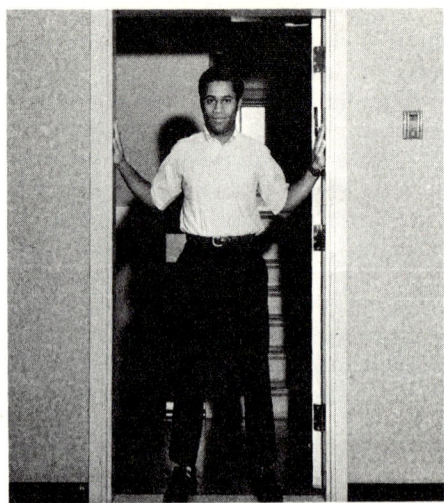

Figure 7. Isometric Exercise

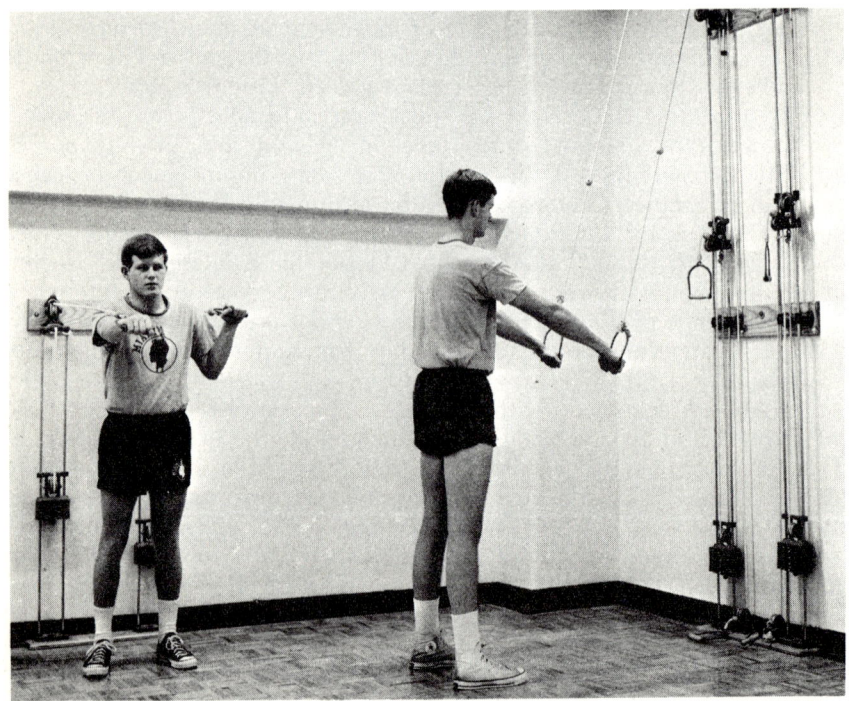

Figure 8. Isotonic Exercise

SOME BASIC UNDERSTANDINGS ABOUT EXERCISE 13

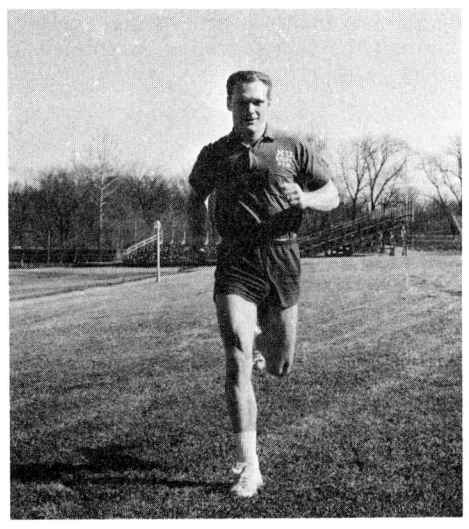

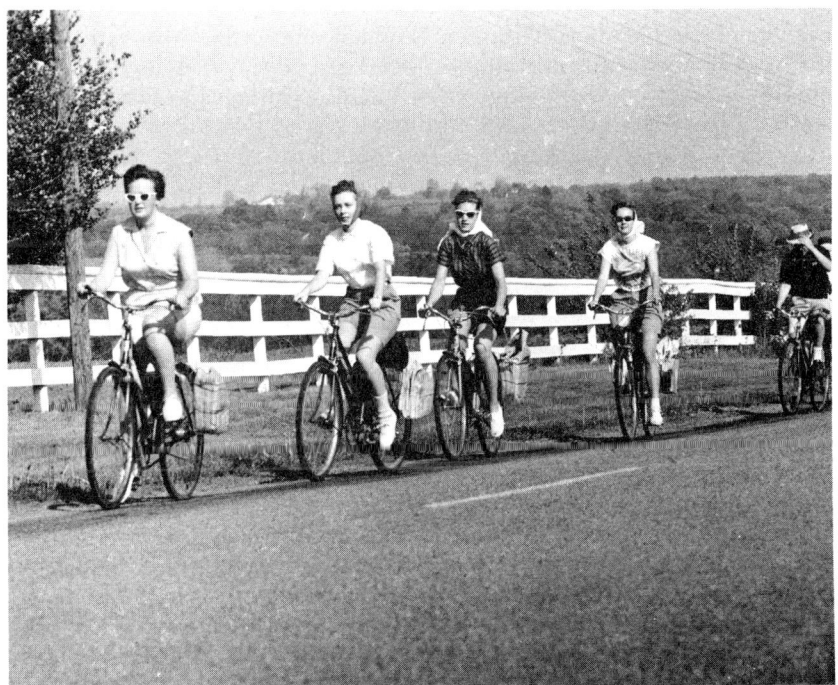

Figure 10. Exercises which Involve Aerobics

Here's a way to measure your physical fitness status. Find out how far you can run *comfortably* in 12 minutes. Then determine your fitness level by checking the distance on this chart:

Distance Covered	Fitness Category
Less than 1 mile	I. Very Poor
1 to 1 1/4 miles	II. Poor
1 to 1 1/2 miles	III. Fair
1 1/2 to 1 3/4 miles	IV. Good
1 3/4 miles or more	V. Excellent

Now you're ready to begin your exercise program. If you prefer to forego the test, start in Category I. Table 1 shows the cycling program and Table 2 applies to running. These charts apply specifically to men but by scaling things down a bit, women can use these also. To use the charts find your category at the left and read across to see what you should do the first week, 2nd week and so on. For those of you in Categories IV or V, you're fit. 30 points a week will keep you that way.

Essentially, aerobics is a type of exercise in which you exert yourself moderately over a period of five minutes, plus. Moderate exercise is a level which you can sustain without becoming so fatigued you are forced to stop in a very short period. This is below the oxygen debt level mentioned earlier. The idea is to elevate your pulse rate to approximately 150 beats per minute and keep it there. After about five minutes of exercise a *training effect* begins. This means that sufficient stress has been placed on your cardiovascular system to cause it to improve its efficiency. The longer you continue exercising beyond five minutes, the more training effect produced. You will recall that in discussing muscle tissue, it was stated that it responds favorably to exercise. This is also true for the cardiovascular system.

Dr. Cooper rates exercises according to the order of their value in producing the training effect. They are: running, swimming, cycling, walking, stationary running, handball, basketball and squash.

Calisthenics. Calisthenics are usually rather formal and they are associated with military training. High school and college athletic teams use this type of activity. Push-ups, jumping jacks and touching the toes, done in unison, are exercises of this type. Generally, calisthenics are in the isotonic category. The Royal Canadian Air Force Physical fitness programs and the President's Council on Physical Fitness booklet "Adult Physical Fitness" include examples of this approach to exercise. Properly conceived, as these programs are, they can be quite effective in maintaining strength and developing *local endurance* and *general endurance*. Flexibility can also be improved. Dr. Cooper, however, would question the value of calisthenics, in producing the *training effect*.

Probably the greatest disadvantage of calisthenics is the matter of motivation. It takes a dedicated person to pursue these rather uninterest-

SOME BASIC UNDERSTANDINGS ABOUT EXERCISE

TABLE 1

AEROBICS CYCLING PROGRAM

CATEGORY I	CATEGORY II	CATEGORY III	DISTANCE (miles)	TIME (mins.)	TIMES a week	POINTS a week
Week	Week					
1st	1st	..	2.0	7:45	5	10
2nd	..	..	2.0	6:45	5	10
3rd	2nd	1st	2.0	6:15	5	10
4th	3rd	..	3.0	11:00	5	15
5th	4th	2nd	3.0	10:00	5	15
6th	5th	3rd	3.0	9:15	5	15
7th	6th	..	4.0	15:00	5	20
8th	..	4th	4.0	13:30	5	20
9th	7th	5th	4.0	12:30	5	20
10th	8th	..	{4.0 / 5.0}	{12:30 / 16:30}	{4 / 1}	21
11th	9th	6th	{4.0 / 5.0}	{12:30 / 16:00}	{3 / 2}	22
12th	..	7th	{4.0 / 6.0}	{12:15 / 19:00}	{3 / 2}	24
13th	10th	..	{4.0 / 6.0}	{12:05 / 18:30}	{3 / 2}	24
14th	11th	8th	{5.0 / 6.0}	{15:30 / 18:30}	{3 / 2}	27
15th	12th	9th	6.0	19:00	5	30
16th	13th	10th	8.0	25:30	4	32

CATEGORIES IV AND V

	DISTANCE	TIME	TIMES a week	POINTS a week
To maintain fitness after completion of conditioning program follow any one of these alternatives:	5.0	15:00-19:59	6	30
	6.0	18:00-23:59	5	30
	8.0	24:00-31:59	4	32
	10.0	30:00-39:59	3	30

Reprinted by permission of M. Evans and Company, Inc., New York, N.Y. Copyright © 1968 Kenneth H. Cooper, M.D. and Kevin Brown.

TABLE 2

AEROBICS RUNNING PROGRAM

CATEGORY I	CATEGORY II	CATEGORY III	DISTANCE (miles)	TIME (mins.)	TIMES a week	POINTS a week
Week	Week					
1st	1st	..	1	13:30	5	10
2nd			1	13	5	10
3rd	2nd	1st	1	12:45	5	10
4th	3rd	..	1	11:45	5	15
5th	4th	2nd	1	11	5	15
6th	5th	3rd	1	10:30	5	15
7th	6th	..	1	9:45	5	20
8th	..	4th	1	9:30	5	20
9th	7th	5th	1	9:15	5	20
10th	8th	..	{1, 1½}	{9 / 16}	{3 / 2}	21
11th	9th	6th	{1, 1½}	{8:45 / 15}	{3 / 2}	21
12th	..	7th	{1, 1½}	{8:30 / 14}	{3 / 2}	24
13th	10th	..	{1, 1½}	{8:15 / 13:30}	{3 / 2}	24
14th	11th	8th	{1, 1½}	{7:55 / 13}	{3 / 2}	27
15th	12th	9th	{1, 1½, 2}	{7:45 / 12:30 / 18}	{2 / 2 / 1}	30
16th	13th	10th	{1½, 2}	{11:55 / 17}	{2 / 2}	31

CATEGORIES IV AND V

To maintain fitness after completion of conditioning program, follow any one of these alternatives:	1	8	6	30
	1	6:30	5	30
	1½	12	4	30
	2	16	3	30

Note: Start program by walking. Then walk/run, or run, as necessary, to meet the changing time goals.

Reprinted by permission of M. Evans and Company, Inc., New York, N.Y. Copyright © 1968 Kenneth H. Cooper, M.D. and Kevin Brown.

ing activities over a long period of time. Many people start such programs only to lose interest after a few days or weeks. There are those, of course, who do persist and gain the benefits of these exercises.

Weight Training. Weight training was formerly referred to as weight lifting. This is a small change on the surface but represents a rather distinct change in practice and philosophy. Weight lifters were the body beautiful devotees of the past. They were more concerned with the size of their biceps, the definition of their muscles and self-admiration in front of a mirror than the more functional aspects of exercise. The term "musclebound" was in vogue in the 1920's and 1930's. Literally it means that an individual had developed so much muscle bulk that he had very restricted movement of the limbs. Although weight lifters did lose some flexibility due to improper use of weights, the musclebound factor was grossly exaggerated. Aspersion was also cast on the intellect of weight lifters. This didn't help their image any either. It's no wonder that for many years college women were afraid of exercising and developing big, bulging muscles.

Modern weight trainers use barbells, plates and various weight-loaded apparatus as a means of keeping fit or in preparation for competition with other enthusiasts. They are proud of their physique and have a healthful regard for their body. Theirs is not the distorted view of the weight lifters of the past. Through stretching their muscles as well as using shortening contraction, they maintain flexibility of joint action.

Here's an example of how you can use weights and retain your flexibility. In doing a curl with a barbell, grasp the barbell with both hands with arms extended in front of your body. The biceps shorten in contraction as you lift the barbell toward your chest. By lowering the barbell all the way until your arms are straight, you stretch your biceps. This prevents your biceps from becoming short and tight and restricting the movement of your arms. Similar examples can be shown with the other muscles of your body.

Weight training has become quite popular among college men. While a considerable amount of equipment is necessary, a vigorous workout can be attained in a fairly short time. Strength in specific muscle groups can be developed rather efficiently. *Local endurance* is enhanced but probably not *general endurance*. Dr. Kenneth Cooper would classify weight training with calisthenics for the same reason—insufficient duration in the activity. No training effect occurs.

College women have not shown much interest in weight training. Their interest in graceful movement through flexibility, and the negativism of the past are important factors in their decision.

Exercise through Sports Participation. While increasing numbers of college men and to some extent college women are participating in isotonics and isometrics, the highest frequency of exercise participation is in sports and games. Strength, endurance, the training effect, flexibility and fun—can all be attained through sports participation. Add to it the

1. Who have greater flexibility, males or females? Explain this from an evolutionary viewpoint.
2. Once atrophy occurs, can the original muscle strength ever be regained?
3. Which form of exercise would you recommend for general body conditioning if you could only select one: isometric or isotonic? Why?
4. How has the American male image changed during the past few decades?

thrill of competition, the satisfying social experiences and the popularity of sports is readily understandable. In any event, you'll have to make your own decision regarding how much and what kind of exercise serves your needs best.

Items for Discussion:

1. Define these terms:
   (a) tonus; (b) overload principle; (c) strength; (d) endurance (local and general); (e) isometrics; (f) isotonics; (g) aerobics.
2. What immediate cardiovascular and respiratory changes occur in your body as you exercise?

Selected Readings

Cooper, Kenneth H. *Aerobics.* New York: Bantam Books. 1968.
Monroe, Keith. "Six Seconds for Exercise." *Reader's Digest.* July, 1959. p. 51.
Smith, Lafayette. "Run For Your Health." *Today's Health.* October, 1964. p. 34.
"Your Muscles: How They Work, Why They Hurt." *Changing Times.* November, 1966. p. 21.

CHAPTER 3

Exercise and Physical Fitness

Physical fitness is a term you see and hear frequently today. What does it mean? *Physical fitness* is maintaining a state of strength and endurance which enables you to carry on your daily activities efficiently and have reserve power at the end of the day to engage in recreational pursuits. You should also be able to meet special challenges which may occur. In emergencies, sudden and unusual demands may be forced upon you. Having sufficient strength, endurance and agility or lack of same may spell the difference between survival and tragedy.[1] This is a minimum goal to be attained and will vary in terms of your own drive for activity. Some of you will be satisfied with a low level of physical fitness while others will seek much higher levels.

You may ask the question, "How do you know when you're physically fit?" If you asked that question to several college students who enjoy high levels of fitness, their answers may vary but essentially they would say this: "When I exercise regularly, I just feel better." "I have more energy than when I'm inactive." "I have a lot of zip and go." "I enjoy my friends and I feel like I'm moving forward most of the time."

From these statements, you will note that part of being fit is having your body well-conditioned and part is a positive attitude toward life. As health educators have known for some time, you can't separate the physical from the mental and social.

These values of physical fitness are valid but quite subjective. There are more tangible results from exercising regularly.

Benefits of Exercise

Quite a few things happen to your body as a direct result of exercise. It was mentioned earlier that muscular *strength* and *endurance* is improved. The strength gain is accompanied by an increase in size of the

---

[1]American Medical Association, *Exercise Fitness,* Chicago: The Association, 1964, p. 1.

muscle. This is called *hypertrophy*. This does not mean that young women need worry about developing masculine builds because of prolonged exercise. College women can develop adequate strength without over-sized muscles.

Another benefit relates to *fatigue*. You not only feel less tired when you exercise regularly, but objective measures of your performance show significant improvement. You can do more push-ups, play more sets of tennis and swim farther when you participate regularly. Your body's resistance to fatigue is the result of more efficient respiratory and cardiovascular function. Your breath rate and heart rate at rest are lowered. Your heart delivers more blood on each pulsation. This means that your heart is doing more work in less time than the untrained heart.

Physical activity is effective in easing *mental tension*. Smashing a handball, a tennis ball or running or swimming a few lengths of a pool can do wonders at pressure-packed final exam time. It's valuable at other tense moments as well.

Exercise is often accompanied by satisfying *social experiences*. "Go where the action is," is the admonition of today's college students. Sports and games are where the action is. It's been said, "If you really want to learn what a person's like, compete with him or her in sports."

There can be great *satisfaction* from exercise. Hayes Jones, U. S. hurdler in the 1962 Olympics, expressed it well after winning his event. "I can't tell you the feeling, the thrill of it. I gave my medal to the kids of Pontiac, Michigan, and it's there now in Pontiac City Hall. It wasn't the medal that mattered, don't you see? It was the experience." A bit of that thrill can be yours whenever you pit yourself against a previous personal record or a fellow student. Whether it's adding another pull up to your previous best or beating your roommate at tennis for the first time, it's a gratifying experience.

Another benefit of exercise is *flexibility*. If you watch the movements of a baby you will quickly see the meaning of the word flexibility. A baby puts his toes in his mouth without any strain. His back is as pliant as a piece of clay. He can curve the bottom of his feet so that he can nearly touch his toes to his heel. Unfortunately, this tremendous suppleness decreases as you grow older. Part of this is due to the increasing density of bones and part is due to mounting restrictions in your movement patterns. As a youngster you ran, jumped, twisted your body, rolled into a ball and continually stretched your muscles. Many of you, however, became less active during adolescence and thus you began to lose some of your flexibility. The loss of flexibility results from failure to move your arms, legs and trunk through a complete range of motion on a regular basis.

The results of the now famous Kraus-Weber tests are dramatic evidence of restricted range of motion or flexibility among American children. The flexibility portion of the test is very simple. It consists of leaning forward and touching your toes, keeping your legs straight while you

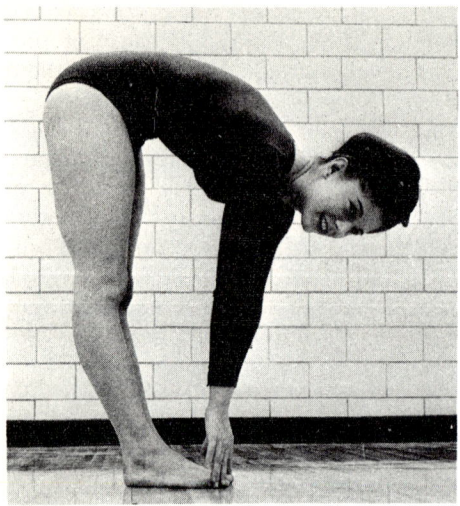

Figure 11. Normal Flexibility

do it (Figure 11). An amazing number of children failed this test. Try it yourself. As you try the test, you may feel some strain in the back of your knees and in the lower part of your back. If you fail the test it means the hamstring muscles located in the back of your upper leg are too short and tight. The same goes for the muscles in your lower back or lumbar region.

Some of the problems related to this kind of lack of flexibility will be discussed in Chapter 6. But what are the positive benefits of flexibility? Improved skill performance in sports is one (Figures 12 and 13). Watch a first baseman digging a low throw out of the dirt. Without flexibility he couldn't manage the "splits" without tearing muscle tissue. Observe the graceful fluid movements of an accomplished dancer. Elongated muscles are much in evidence. Ever wonder why children are so good at the hulahoop? Flexibility is the answer.

Dancing to today's pop music calls for extensive pelvic gyrations. You have to be flexibility to be skillful at this type of dancing. If you're inhibited or tight-muscled, you'll look awkward and feel more so.

Another result of being flexible is that you'll present a better appearance. Your posture or bearing is definitely related to the tautness of your muscles.

Physical education instruction for college women places more emphasis on flexibility than do programs for college men. Cultural patterns, however, would dictate that after college women become physically inactive sooner than men. Child-rearing and home making are definite factors causing this. Sedentary living results in loss of flexibility and thus needs to be on continuing concern for both men and women during college and the years that follow.

EXERCISE AND PHYSICAL FITNESS 21

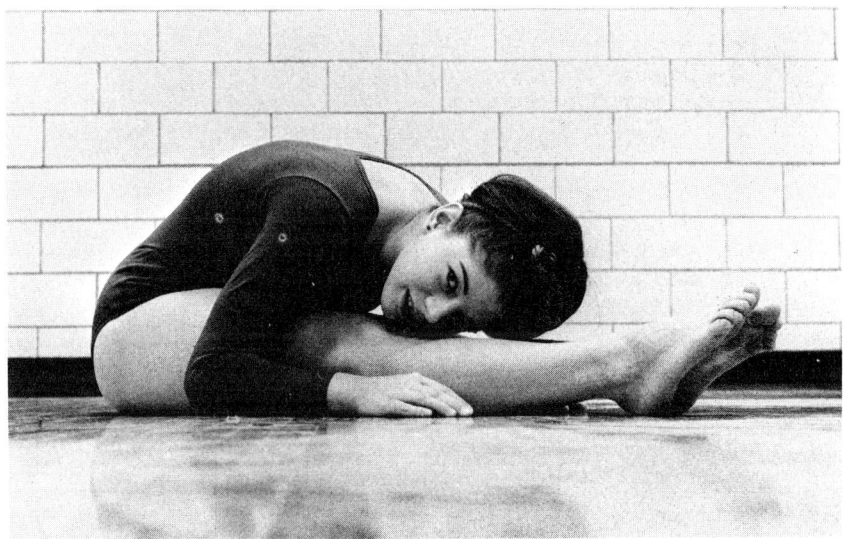

Figure 12

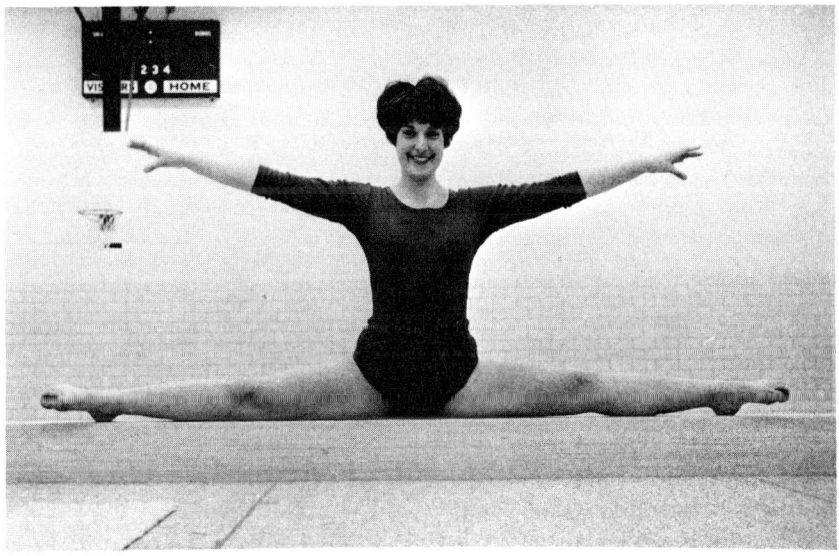

Figure 13
Unusual Flexibility

> 1. Is it possible to increase muscle strength without increasing muscle size (hypertophy)?
> 2. What physical benefits can be derived from the forms of dance currently popular among our youth?
> 3. What do you understand by the term "physical fitness"? How can you tell if you're physically fit?
> 4. Is physical fitness really necessary in this day of mechanization and automation? Do you really care if you are 'physically fit'?

Can you expect to live longer if you exercise? The important thing is not how long you live but how *well* you live. The quality of living is vastly more important than the quantity of living. The American Medical Association, however, states that, "As far as can be determined at the present time, the study of life histories of those who maintain a relatively higher degree of fitness through the nature of their work or through other activities seems to indicate that they suffer less degenerative disease and probably live longer than those who follow a sedentary life."[2]

ITEMS FOR DISCUSSION:
1. What is physical fitness?
2. How do you know when you're physically fit?
3. What are the benefits of exercise?

SELECTED READINGS

FLETCHER, COLIN. "I've Rediscovered Walking." *Reader's Digest*. March, 1963. p. 139.

HARMOUNT, JAMES GODFREY. "55 Million Cyclists Can't Be Wrong." *Today's Health*. October, 1964. p. 32.

STEINHAUS, ARTHUR H. *How To Keep Fit and Like It*. Chicago: The Dartnell Corporation. 1957.

---

[2]*Ibid*. p. 5.

CHAPTER 4

Selecting Exercises For Your Needs

Having developed some understandings about exercise and physical fitness, you need some guidelines for selecting activities. You need answers to the questions, "How much exercise do I need?" "How often should I exercise?" "On what basis should I pick activities?"

The answer to the first question is relatively simple. The prime basis for your selection should be enjoyment. History tells us that if you are going to exercise now and in the future the experience must be largely a pleasurable one. Not too many college students, can discipline themselves to engage in vigorous activity on a regular basis if they feel that it is painful, unpleasant drudgery which they endure for the side benefits.

Since there is such a wide range of activities to select from, satisfaction and enjoyment can be attained by virtually everyone. A plus factor in gaining pleasure is having adequate skill in the activity. The dub golfer may find the game quite frustrating. The novice tennis player who spends more time chasing the ball than hitting it may find little satisfaction. The inexperienced weight trainer who through improper technique drops a barbell on his foot finds this highly undesirable. The beginning swimmer who misjudges his ability and becomes frightened in deep water is not developing a lifetime love of the water.

As a college student, there are opportunities for you to develop skills in a whole host of sports and games through instruction in your college physical education program. Many students select their course in terms of ease of scheduling rather than through intelligent decisions based on their physical, mental and social needs.

College and university departments of physical education have your needs in mind in planning the sequence of courses. These include such things as physical fitness testing programs so you can appraise your status. Also offered are sports orientation courses which involve classroom work or actual participation, on an introductory basis, in a wide variety of sports. In addition, many programs have their activities classified according to their contributions to your physical, mental and social needs. Thus, you have vigorous team activities: combatives for men such as wrestling, aquatic activities, conditioning courses which include running and weight training, physical fitness-body mechanics for women, and individual and dual sports such as golf, tennis and badminton. Some universities, in an attempt to increase your participation in college and after graduation, are including classroom instruction in the "why" of exercise and sports involvement. These college physical education departments feel that if you understand what happens to you physiologically, psychologically and socially you will be motivated to make exercise a part of your everyday living. This is in agreement with the purposes of this book.

Let's assume that you were free to tailor-make your own exercise program. Here are some suggestions to guide you in your selection of activities:

1. Remember that you're selecting activities for the present and the future.
2. Unless you develop desirable *habits* and *attitudes* toward exercise, now, your activity level will drop sharply and decline to a minimum after graduation.
3. Availability of facilities is a factor to consider. For example, handball is a fine activity for men to learn and enjoy in college, and modern dance provides worthwhile experiences for college women; but opportunities for participation after college are somewhat limited.
4. Some activities require high levels of fitness to be safe and enjoyable. Wrestling for men and gymnastics for women are sports of this type.
5. Remember that some sports have greater social potential than others.
6. Exercising regularly, at least three times per week, and in moderate doses is the best way to attain maximum benefits.
7. A variety of activities is needed for maintenance of strength and endurance in different muscle groups.
8. Determine what you hope to achieve and then plan your sports and exercise program.

Now let's consider specific activities and how they contribute to your needs.

Running and Jogging and Walking

Running, of course, is a very vigorous mode of exercise. It is an excellent conditioner for your legs and promotes cardiovascular and respiratory efficiency. Slow down the pace and you become a jogger. The book, "Jogging" by William J. Bowerman, Track Coach, University of Oregon, and W. E. Harris, M.D., has aroused great interest among the U. S. populace.[1] Men and women, businessmen and housewives collec-

---

[1] William J. Bowerman and W. E. Harris, "Jogging," New York: Grosset and Dunlap. 1967.

tively, are logging thousands of miles along our country's highways and byways. By picking your jogging course carefully, you can combine exercise with beautiful scenery and pleasant surroundings. From a practical point of view it is good to get off the concrete highway and onto turf. Running on hard surfaces can be irritating to your feet, knees and leg muscles.

Walking seems like such a mild activity you may not consider it worthwhile exercise. If you're on a large university campus, you may recall, however, that each fall you have to become accustomed to scurrying between classes from building to building. Brisk walking does the same for you as running and jogging. It just takes more of it.

Swimming

Swimming has a range of strenuousness similar to the running, jogging, walking sequence. It can be used to efficiently develop the "training effect." Swimming also contributes to your arm and shoulder strength and local endurance. Water as a sedative or relaxing agent has been used for thousands of years. Development of your competency in swimming provides you with basis for safe participation in a number of aquatic activities such as boating, fishing, water skiing, surfing and sailing. Contrary to a popular belief among college students, swimming does not increase susceptibility to the common cold.

Sports and Games

A considerable number of sports and games are available to you as college students. Some sports like golf and bowling do more for your social success than your muscles, or your cardiovascular system. Don't be misled by the statement, "I'll wait until I'm too old to do anything else and then I'll learn to play golf or bowl." There's ample evidence that most outstanding performers in any sport learned the skills at a young age. Even if you don't aspire to be a champion, you'll learn better now and enjoy participation more than if you wait five or ten years.

Other sports available to you, like field hockey for women and soccer for men, are active team games with limited carry-over value. Their merit lies in your satisfaction in performing as a member of a group. And they are good tension valves. As you become immersed in a rugged game of this sort, your problems are submerged. This is also an excellent opportunity to channel aggressive behavior into an acceptable pathway. After sitting in class for several hours, charging up and down a field in hot pursuit of a soccer ball or hockey ball can be a most exhilarating experience.

Weight Training

Weight training may suggest to you huge men struggling with massive barbells but this type of equipment can be used in a variety of ways. A barbell which is a bar 5 or 6 feet long, and a dumbbell, a bar 10 to 14 inches in length, and iron plates constitute the basic equipment. The plates range in weight from 1¼ pounds to 50 pounds and act as the resistance which is used in the "overload principle." With such a variation of graduated resistance available, you can gain strength, improve local endurance and increase your muscle size, according to your needs.

If you're recovering from a muscle injury or a fractured bone which results in weakened muscles, you can use weights for therapeutic purposes. By starting with a light weight and gradually adding weight and repetitions you gradually regain normal function of your muscles. Another value of weight training is that it can provide you with the means of changing your bodily appearance. It's amazing what confidence comes with the development of well-defined muscles. You feel stronger, look stronger and feel you can handle yourself in any situation. Despite the lessened physical demands of today's living, the possession of muscular strength is a source of great satisfaction.

Weight training too can be an effective means of weight control. Short periods of lifting will aid in gaining weight and long periods of effort can result in weight reduction.

A challenge is inherent in weight training as you strive for higher levels of achievement. Meeting a challenge is psychologically stimulating. And weight training as done by college men is an excellent medium for developing friendships.

Isometrics

You will recall that in Chapter 2 it was stated that isometrics is an effective way of developing strength. So you must decide in what muscle groups you need strength. Some college women have difficulty controlling a tennis racket, a golf club or bowling ball because of insufficient hand and arm strength. Isometrics is a quick and easy answer to the problem. For best results your isometric exercise must closely approximate the position used in the particular sport. If you plan to improve your hand and arm strength for the forehand drive in tennis, for example, your body and arm must be in a position similar to the forehand drive as you execute the isometric exercise.

Evaluating your Exercise Program

Having selected a number of different means of exercising how do you know you're achieving your goals? Regarding social outcomes, satisfaction, release of tension and fun or pleasure, you'll have to make

SELECTING EXERCISES FOR YOUR NEEDS 27

your own subjective appraisal. Even though you're making the judgment yourself without the use of precise scientific instruments your evaluation is certainly valid. When you feel great because of a regular exercise, you're well aware of it. It's a definite plus factor in your daily effectiveness.

There are other more precise methods of appraising your status.

Physical Examination. It's a wise practice to have a complete medical evaluation annually, but particularly before you embark on an exercise program (Figure 14). The examination should include an evaluation of your cardiovascular efficiency. This includes appraisal of your heart action at rest, immediately after exercise, and at intervals up to six minutes after exercise. By listening to your heart, your physician can determine how you respond to exercise and how long it takes to recover to its normal resting status. An electrocardiograph test is also highly recommended as a further evaluation tool. Having a record of your heart action is useful as a basis for comparisons throughout your lifetime.

Your physician may also discover some conditions affecting your muscles or joints which would be aggravated by certain kinds of exercises.

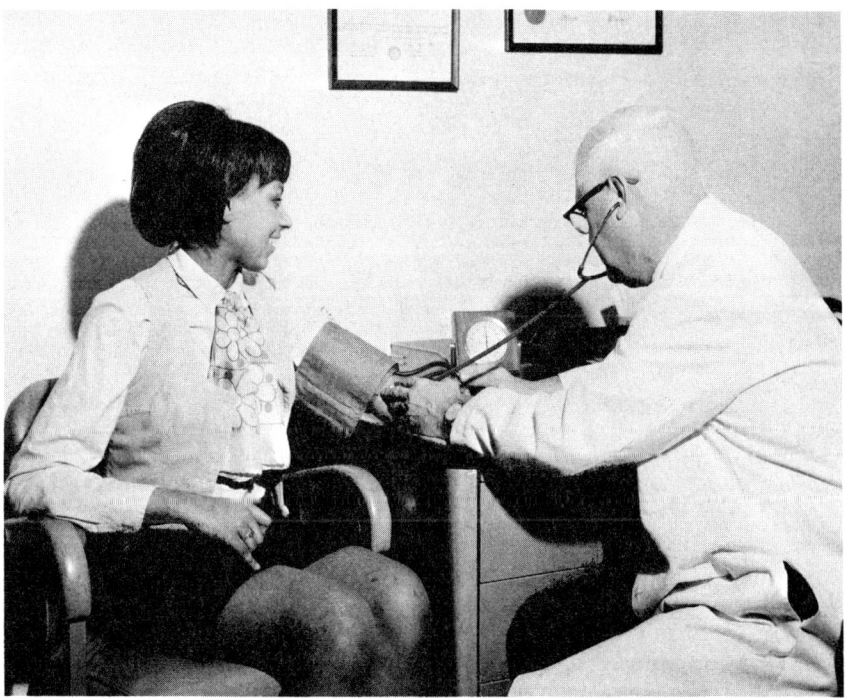

Figure 14. Physical Examination

Your Own Cardiovascular Test. If you're interested in performing your own cardiovascular test, you can do so quite easily (Figure 15). First, take your pulse rate while you're in a standing position. This is done by placing the finger tips of your right hand against your neck just below the jaw line on the left side of your face. Take your pulse for 30 seconds and multiply by two. Then, run in place for two minutes, lifting your feet at least eight inches from the floor. Take your pulse rate immediately after exercise. It will be 120-160 beats per minute. Take it again at two minutes, four minutes and six minutes. If you're in good condition, your pulse rate six minutes after exercise should be what it was before exercise. By recording the results of this test and retaking it periodically, you can chart your progress in becoming physically fit. This test is appropriate for both college men and women, although

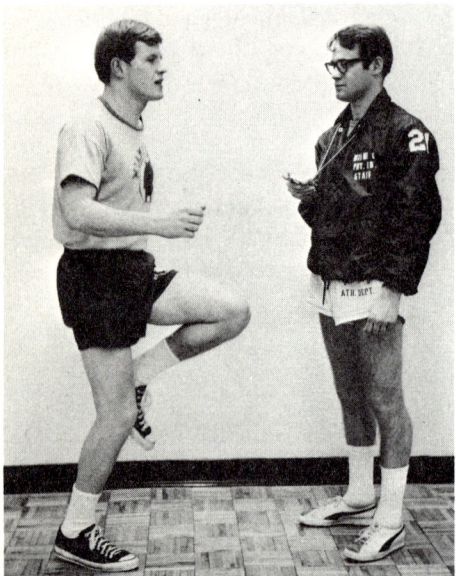

Figure 15. Cardiovascular Test

women will have a somewhat longer recovery period. The average heart rate for men at rest (sitting or lying down) is 78, and 84 beats per minute for women. In the standing position, as used in the above test, the pulse rate will average 15 beats per minute higher than for the sitting position.

Other Measures of Progress. For sports like swimming and running, you can easily determine your progress by measuring the distance traversed and the time it takes to do this. The book "Aerobics" contains well-defined progressions which are easy to interpret.[2]

---
[2]Cooper, Kenneth, *op. cit.*

1. Jay Sylvester, a college freshman, was overheard saying "all forms of exercise are painful; yet you claim that the prime basis of my selection should be enjoyment. I guess that eliminates all types for me!" How would you challenge him?
2. What is the relationship between body type and the selection of exercises? (eg. would you recommend jogging or swimming for a fat person?)
3. Your father has suddenly developed an interest in exercise—apparently he attended a lecture on fitness delivered by an "expert". What advise will you give him (on preparing to exercise, forms of exercise, and duration of his program)?

Progressions in weight training and calisthenics are recorded in terms of the amount of weight or resistance and the number of repetitions.

Items for Discussion:
1. On what basis should you select your exercise activities?
2. How do the following contribute to your exercise needs?
   (a) Running, jogging and walking;
   (b) Swimming;
   (c) Sports and games, weight training;
   (d) Isometrics

Selected Readings

BOWERMAN, WILLIAM J. and HARRIS, W. E. "Jogging." New York: Grosset and Dunlap. 1967.

FLINT, MARILYN. "Selecting Exercises." *Journal of Health, Physical Education, and Recreation.* February, 1964. p. 19.

IRWIN, THEODORE. "Don't Be A Weekend Athlete." *Today's Health.* July, 1966. p. 46.

President's Council on Physical Fitness. *Adult Fitness: A Program for Men and Women.* Washington, D. C. Government Printing Office. 1963.

Royal Canadian Air Force Exercise Plans for Physical Fitness. *Pocket Books, Inc.* New York, 1962.

CHAPTER 5

Consumer Information About Exercise Equipment

Through magazines, newspapers and television you are being constantly bombarded with information about a multitude of products and services. Currently, exercise and physical fitness equipment and services are receiving much attention from ad-men and marketing experts. This means decisions, decisions, decisions for you.

Equipment

You'll be exposed to terms like Relaxorcisor, Exergene, Exercycle, Tone-o-matic, and York barbells. In evaluating exercise equipment, you must first discover its specific purpose and design. Firsthand examination is best, of course, but you may have to rely on pictures and descriptions. Try to figure out the exercise principle which the equipment employs. If the instructions state that you're to press or push against something and there's little movement involved, it's isometrics. The resistance to movement may be in the form of springs as in the Tone-a-lator. Some devices, like the Exergene, uses the friction of rope on pulleys inside a cylinder to provide an isometric exercise. A simple adjustment of the pulley arrangement enables the user to reduce friction and move through a range of motion as in an isotonic exercise. Thus, you can get isometric and isotonic exercise with the same piece of equipment.

There are a number of exercise bicycles on the market. They use friction devices, usually a roller which presses against the tire, to provide varying degrees of resistance to your pedaling. Some have speedometers so you can tell how fast and far you have cycled. Cycling, whether stationery or on a regular bike, is excellent exercise for your legs but is less effective for the arms and upper body.

Be wary of exercise bicycles which have an electric motor which does the work while you watch your feet go around. This is a passive exercise and produces little change in your fitness. There are basic physiological principles operating here. To develop strength and/or endurance, there must be active contraction of your muscles. In fact, your muscles must be taxed beyond normal usage for positive results to occur. This is the "overload" principle which was discussed in Chapter 2.

Some of the exercise bicycle manufacturers have discovered the poor results from passive exercise and have redesigned their equipment to provide resistance to the leg movement.

Since the matter of how much exercise is always a major concern, "exercise monitors" are being added to bicycles. This device tells you how much effort is required and provides precise measures of periods of exercise and rest. As a college student the price tag will alarm you, but as a future executive, professional man, or wife of same, you should be aware of the more scientific approaches to exercise.

Another type of apparatus which you should know about is the massage machine. It may be in the form of a vibrating mechanism in which metal parts oscillate against your body. Another type uses belts which vibrate at a high rate of speed. These machines are purported to make the pounds melt away. They do have the beneficial effect of increasing circulation through the massaging action. And they certainly give you a pleasant sensation. Their ability to help you lose weight is very questionable, however, and they can do nothing for your muscle tone or conditioning.

Another item which is related to weight reduction is sweat clothing. It may be sold under the more exotic name of suana suit, but the technique employed is the same. A non-porous material like plastic or nylon is used in a two-piece outfit: jacket and trousers. The suit is snug-fitting around the neck, waist, wrists and ankles. A short workout in a warm room and you perspire profusely. If you're doing this to lose weight, you will lose; but this is a water loss which you'll probably regain quickly if you succumb to your developing thirst. Worn for a short period of time there are no harmful effects from the use of a suit of this type. If you feel good as a result of perspiring, this can be worthwhile for you. There is danger, however, if you exercise violently for long periods particularly in hot weather. Dehydration and a rise in body temperature results. Heat exhaustion, a serious menace to your health, can be the next step. Under severe conditions, this can be fatal. Athletic coaches, especially football coaches, are alerted to this condition during pre-season practice in the hot month of August. Here are some hot weather exercise hints suggested by the American Medical Association:[1]

1. Work out during cooler morning and early evening hours in hot weather.
2. Acclimate yourself to hot weather activity by carefully graduated amounts of exercise.
3. If you work out for an hour or more, plan to rest for 15 to 30 minutes at the end of the hour's exercise.

---

[1]The American Medical Association, "Tips on Athletic Training, VIII," Chicago: The Association, 1966, p. 6.

4. Wear clothing that is white to reflect heat and wear brief, loose clothing to permit heat to escape. Your clothing should also be permeable to moisture to allow heat loss by perspiration.
5. Consume salt and water to maintain body fluids.
6. Remember that high air temperature and high humidity, not the sun, are the crucial factors. These prevent your body from maintaining normal temperature through perspiration. Heat exhaustion can occur in the shade.

The designers of electronic equipment are not to be left out of the exercise field. This equipment is being promoted as "effortless exercisors." Basically, they are gadgets which have a transistorized power supply. Wires which end in padded, plastic squares are attached to the machine. To use the apparatus, you moisten the plastic pads and place them on the muscles you wish to stimulate. By turning a dial on the machine, electric current streams through the wire to the pads. The current causes your muscles to jump into action. Your muscles contract either mildly or vigorously depending on the strength of current. Used as directed, the muscles are exercised, but if you fail to moisten the pads thoroughly or place them improperly you receive painful electrical impulses. The whole operation takes considerable time. If you're gadget-minded you may like this type of equipment, but there are more enjoyable ways to tone your muscles. The benefits to fitness of these devices, moreover, is unproven.

Remember, you can select forms of exercise which require few or no exercise devices. If these contrivances are your only means to exercise, use them; but be sure you get what you pay for. Here are some consumer guides for you as you select exercise equipment now and in the future:

1. As with any product, compare cost among competitive items.
2. Determine quality of materials and workmanship. Will it hold up under the strain of daily use?
3. Analyze it to discover the physiological principle used. Does it favor isometrics or isotonics?
4. How versatile is the equipment? Can you develop strength and endurance with it? Will it also improve your flexibility?
5. Determine what body parts it develops. Is it good for arms but does little for legs? Is it useful in total body development?
6. What are the space requirements for the apparatus? Can you use it in your room in the dorm?
7. Does the equipment take a special floor covering such as link tire mats for barbells? Your dorm counselor and fellow students may object to the damage to the tile floor and the noise weights create.
8. Guard against a device which is promoted as one which requires no effort on your part for fitness development.
9. Remember that your college physical education instructor is a good

resource person in both planning exercise programs and selecting equipment.

Health Clubs

Men's athletic clubs and the YMCA and YWCA have provided exercise facilities for many years. The newest thing on the American scene are rather plush exercise emporiums known variously as Health Spas, Slenderella or Silhouette. They are designed to appeal to both men and women. According to the Spas' management, this is exercise at its luxurious best. The services offered are many and varied (Figure 16). Figure contouring salon for ladies, mechanical massage and spot reducing, mechanical body re-proportioning machines, turkish steam room, individual mild and progressive exercise programs, infrared sauna rooms, mild, progressive refirming apparatus, ultra-violet beauty ray sun booths, patented electrical reducing machines, oil of eucalyptus inhalation room, large swimming pool, magic profile facial machines, hydra-swirl mineral pool. Under the direction of a professional staff using this equipment,

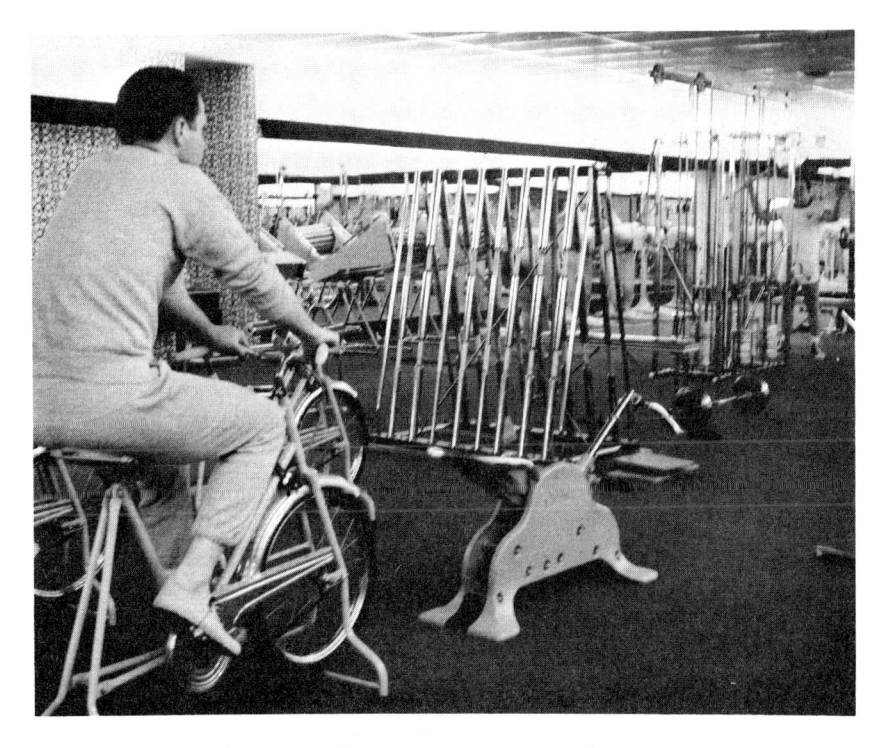

Figure 16 Exercise Equipment at the Spa

the literature indicates the following will result: gain weight, have more fun, more energy, toning, increase circulation, acquire suppleness, better appearance, lose inches, firming, lift, firm, develop bust line, lose weight, improve endurance, reproportion your body, relax and have more pep. In addition you can have a gourmet delight of special health foods in the sumptuous clubroom.

What are you buying when you join the group at the Spa? Essentially, you're paying someone to provide your motivation to exercise. The pleasant surroundings, the maze of equipment and the sedative effects of heat are used to convince you that you can get "optimum results with a minimum of effort." Optimum results implies improved strength and endurance. As you now know, this does take effort. The equipment necessary for maximum benefits is provided in the Spa. Like most things, you get out of an exercise program what effort you put into it.

Exercising at the Spa can certainly firm up some long unused muscles, but reapportionment of your figures, ladies, is a rather extravagant claim. Belt machines and vibrators are not very effective reducers.

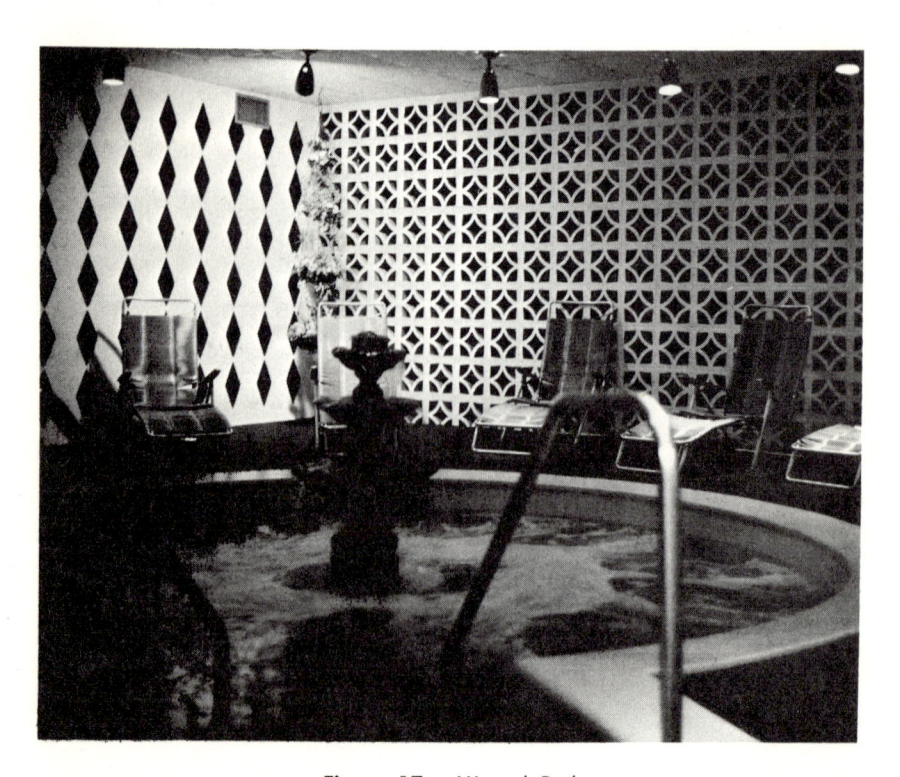

Figure 17. Mineral Bath

1. What type of exercise does a 'weight reducing' belt represent? How effective is this for weight reduction?
2. What role do electric 'vibrators' play in a weight-reducing program?
3. How effective are sauna baths in the long term maintenance of a constant body weight?
4. Middle-aged people often eat less than they did in previous years, yet, still continue to gain weight. How is this possible?

Regular, moderate exercise and reduced caloric intake along with the advice of your physician is a better answer.

If you're seeking relaxation, it can be yours at the Health Spa. Heat in various forms is the medium for reducing your tension. The source of heat in the desert-dry heat room is infrared elements. This is heat without moisture. The sauna bath also provides dry heat. Heated rocks develop a room temperature of 160°-220° at 5 per cent-10 per cent humidity.

The Turkish steam room employs moist heat, 110°-120° with 100 per cent humidity. The so-called mineral baths are really whirlpools large enough to accommodate several people at one time (Figure 17). Jets of air entering the bath below the water level provide a gentle massaging action. This is very beneficial in soothing muscle aches and pains. Some Spas have a small swimming pool with a water temperature of 85° to 90° which also provides a sedative effect.

Health Spas certainly appeal to college-educated men and women. If, in the future, you find it difficult to find the time and place for exercise elsewhere, the Health Spas may fulfill your need.

Items for Discussion:
1. What should you know before purchasing exercise equipment?
2. What are Health Spas and what do they offer?

Selected Readings

Higdon, Hal. "What You Should Know About Saunas," *Today's Health*. March, 1967. p. 20.

CHAPTER 6

Exercise and Special Health Problems

While exercise makes a significant and positive contribution to your overall health, it can also be used in preventing certain health problems from occuring.

Exercise and Posture

Maintenance of good posture can be achieved through an exercise program which emphasizes correct postural habits and balanced muscular development. Basically, your goal is to have good alignment with ease and flexibility (Figure 18). Push the top of your head towards the sky when you're standing or sitting. This will help you to have your body segments poised one above the other. Since each person is constructed somewhat differently in terms of the skeletal and muscle systems, the general posture standards must be applied to each individual. Your physical education instructor will help you to gain a concept of what is good posture for you.

Problems related to muscular imbalance usually affect your posture in two areas of your body; the shoulder-chest region and the low back-abdominal section (Figure 19).

Round Shoulders. The shoulder-chest problem is called thoracic kyphosis or more simply, round shoulders. The causes are either habitual forward slumping of the shoulders; or short, tight pectoral (chest) muscles. In either case, the back is bowed and the chest appears to be depressed. A balanced exercise program which gives equal emphasis to movements which move the arms forward and those which move the arms and shoulders backward, is a preventive measure. Being aware of the proper position of the shoulders and chest is important also. The rigid, military-like position with your shoulders forced back is not recommended. It is not a relaxed posture and is an exaggeration of the desired objective.

It is important to know that round shoulders is not a serious problem from the physical health standpoint. Contrary to what used to be be-

EXERCISE AND SPECIAL HEALTH PROBLEMS 37

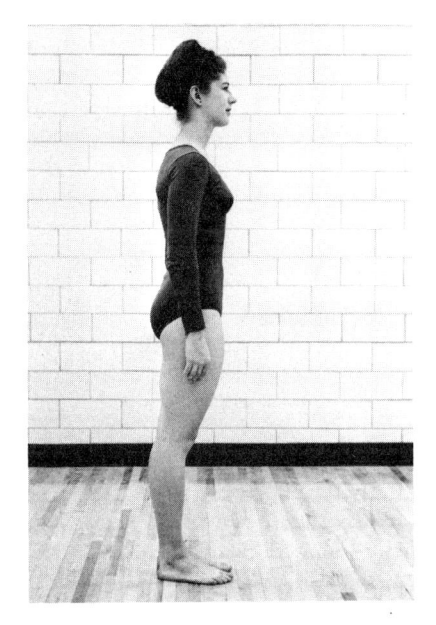

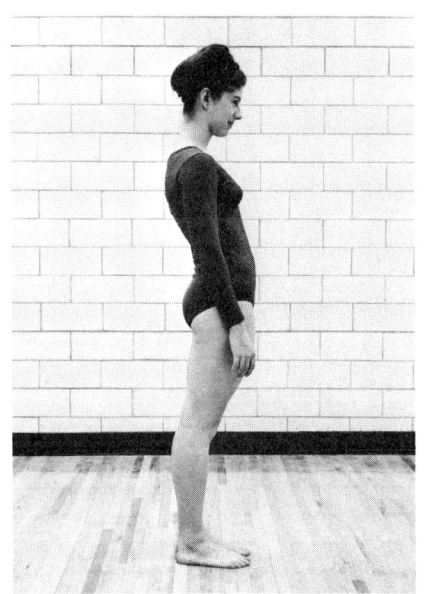

Figure 18. Good Posture

Figure 19. Poor Posture

lieved, round shoulders do not result in impaired breathing or restricted visceral functioning. At least, little scientific evidence exists to support this contention.

Low Back Pain. The low back-abdominal problem is becoming more common among the adult population in the U. S. It's on the increase for college men and women. Low-back syndrome is the term orthopedic physicians use to describe this condition. A dull ache in the small of the back is the way the sufferer refers to it. The exact causes require the evaluation of a physician. Sometimes the cartilaginuous pad, or disc between the lumbar vertebrae, is damaged or congenitally deformed. More often the problem is a muscular one. It is not caused by a "weak back" as many people think but by muscular imbalance. The muscular imbalance develops as the following sequences of events occur.

As you reach adulthood you tend to be less active. The abdominal muscles are among the first to be affected. Flabby abdominal muscles, or ptosis, develops. This is characterized by a protruding abdomen. In extreme cases the visceral contents shift forward and the individual must lean back at the waist with the upper body to maintain body balance.

The same thing occurs during pregnancy for women and accounts for low back pain during that period. Over-eating and high heels magnify the problem. Muscular imbalance occurs as your back muscles in a sense, overpower the weakened abdominals. Leaning backward with the upper body causes increased curve in the lumbar or lower back region to occur. This is known as hyperextension and is accompanied by a strain on the ligaments and sometimes the vertebrae themselves. The back muscles become short and tight, because they are contracting more than usual. When your back muscles become fatigued from overwork, they may go into spasm. A spasm is a powerful, sustained contraction and is most painful. You've probably had a spasm or cramp in your calf muscle. The pain which is associated with low back syndrome is usually caused by these muscle spasms.

To avoid this condition you must do two things: (1) maintain a firm flat abdomen, and (2) retain flexibility in your back muscles. Exercises to accomplish this can be built into your exercise program. An excellent exercise for your abdominals is the following isometric exercise.

Try it first while you're lying on your back. Later you will be able to do it while you are standing or sitting. It's done like this: Draw in your tummy and try to press it against your spinal column. Don't breathe in, just pull in your abdominals. Hold for six seconds. Contract your gluteal muscles at the same time. The gluteal muscles are the ones you sit on. By contracting them at the same time you contract the abdominals, you tend to flatten your back. This will help to avoid excessive curve in the low back area.

A word of caution: do not hold your breath. You may cut off oxygen supply to your brain and get dizzy or faint. To keep from holding your breath, try singing or whistling.

After a little practice, you will be able to make your abdominal wall quite concave. By doing this exercise just once or twice a day, you will be able to maintain good tonus in your abdominals.

There are two simple exercises which help you to keep your back flexible. In the first one you assume a back-lying position. Flex your right leg and bring your knee toward your chest. Put both hands on your knee and pull gently toward your chest. Keep your left leg straight and on the floor. Repeat the exercise with the left leg. Then bring both knees to the chest at the same time. Use your hands to exert some pressure again.

The second exercise is done from a position on your back with your arms extended above your head. Come to a sitting position and exhale slowly as you try to touch your toes. Keep your legs together and keep them straight as you attempt to touch your toes. Do not force the movement, but try to relax as much as possible. Slide your hands down the front of your legs as far as you can, without undue strain. You will be stretching your back muscles and the muscles in back of your legs. Hold this position for a few seconds. Slide your hands back to your knees and relax. Then try it again. Conclude the exercise by going back to the backlying position with the arms overhead. This will help to stretch your abdominal muscles and cause them to relax. Repeat the exercise twice daily.

EXERCISE AND SPECIAL HEALTH PROBLEMS

As your back muscles and your leg muscles become longer, you'll find the strain will diminish. It is best for the sake of comfort to avoid doing this exercise within one hour of a meal. Remember, relaxation is the key. Don't force it. This is a Yoga exercise and the Yoga approach to exercise emphasizes slow, easy movements rather than quick, violent ones.

Foot Problems

When man began to wear shoes and later built concrete floors and sidewalks, he wasn't being kind to his feet. The shoes immediately restricted the motion of his toes and reduced the flexibility of his whole foot. The unyielding concrete provides a spine-jolting shock with each step. Individuals who are born without arms and hands provide ample evidence of the great potential for skilled movements we all possess. They learn to type with their toes, sew, play cards and most of the other tasks people usually perform with their hands and fingers.

Remember, muscles respond to exercise and fade away from disuse. Your feet are no exception. As your feet muscles weaken, fallen arches, loss of function and pain follow. Excess poundage (overweight) is a contributing factor.

Here are some tips for good foot health:
1. Take off your shoes whenever possible and curl up your feet and wiggle your toes.
2. Run barefooted in the sand. Dig in with your toes and drive forward.
3. Rise up on your toes, with your soles turned in, several times a day.
4. Put a towel on the floor and crumple it up with your toes.
5. Pick up marbles or other objects with your toes.
6. Wear properly fitted shoes.

These suggestions like the exercises for postural deviations are intended to forestall problems. If you develop malfunctions which relate to muscles, bones or joints, see your physician. He may refer you to the medical specialist who deals with this type of malady, the orthopedist. The orthopedic specialist may prescribe therapeutic exercises to eliminate your problem.

Good Body Mechanics and Exercise

Body mechanics are concerned with efficient use of the body with particular reference to the muscular and skeletal systems. Stooping, lifting, walking and sports skills are all movements which can be injurious if done incorrectly. There are also body mechanics procedures which apply to all the types of exercises mentioned earlier. By observing good practices you gain positive results from your exercise while minimizing the poor effects. Our first consideration is the preparation for muscular activity.

Warmup. You will recall that muscle tissue is elastic. It will stretch, but, of course, there are limitations. A cold muscle is less elastic than a warm one and thus more prone to injury. So a warmup prior to vigorous exercise is highly advisable. You can warmup artificially by standing under a warm shower for three to five minutes. Researchers have found this to be an effective method. The more conventional way is to perform calisthenics slowly and gradually until you are perspiring freely. By this time your body temperature has been elevated about one degree and you're ready for more strenuous action.

Flexibility Exercises. If you plan your warmup activity wisely, you can include flexibility exercises and further prevent the possibility of injury. A stretched or elongated muscle is less prone to being torn when called into play than a short, tight one. It's a good idea to stretch the muscles which are most involved in the sport or exercise you are about to perform. Be sure and do the stretching slowly and gently. Do not use quick movements. Watch the divers, gymnasts or track athletes on your college teams as they do stretching exercises, and you'll get the idea.

If you develop a muscle spasm or your muscles become sore from too much exercise, stretching them will cause them to relax and the pain will subside. This is based upon a physiological principle—the law of *reciprocal innervation.* When you contract your biceps as in lifting a suitcase, nerve impulses go to your opposing or antagonistic muscle, the triceps, causing it to relax. This enables you to have a smooth, coordinated movement rather than a tight, awkward one. When you stretch your muscle, the same thing happens. The muscle in spasm receives stimuli, stops contracting, and tension is reduced. You've probably used this method of reducing tension and pain without knowing how it worked. If you've ever had a cramp or spasm in the calf of your leg, you got relief by pulling the top of your foot toward your head. This stretched the gastrocnemius muscle and it relaxed.

Exercises to Avoid. Certain exercises violate principles of good body mechanics and for general use should be avoided. Exercises which cause hyperextension or exaggerated curve of the lower back (arching) are in this category. While it is true that the varsity gymnasts and divers, both men and women, are required to develop great range of motion in their back and trunk, most people can't tolerate much hyperextension. Exercises which cause hyperextension include: (1) double leg lifts from a backlying position, (2) situps with the legs straight, and, (3) the arching swan in the prone position.

Another exercise to avoid is deep knee bends. This puts great pressure on the knee joint. Performing this movement while holding a barbell or other weight adds to the strain on the joint. A quarter or half-knee bend will accomplish the desired results of strengthening the front thigh or quadriceps muscles without the ill effects.

EXERCISE AND SPECIAL HEALTH PROBLEMS

Your physical education instructor is a good person to consult regarding questionable exercises.

Exercise and Cardiovascular Conditions

The term, cardiovascular, refers to your heart, veins and arteries. As noted earlier, the cardiovascular system becomes more efficient with regular exercise. There's a preventive aspect here, too. The American Heart Association and prominent physicians like Dr. Dudley Allen White are convinced that regular exercise throughout your life reduces your risk of heart disease. In addition, the beneficial effects of exercise give you an edge over the sedentary individual if you do have a heart attack. You're more likely to survive and more likely to recover from it. In response to exercise your heart becomes stronger and beats slower. It does more work with less effort. Not only does your heart pump more blood with each pulsation but your heart develops additional *capillarization*. Capillarization involves the formation of increased pathways through which blood can flow. This is important in providing adequate blood supply to all parts of the heart. If you suffer a *coronary heart attack* this means that a coronary vessel has become blocked with a blood clot or *embolus*. The increased capillarization resulting from regular exercise becomes vital to the repair of the damaged portion of the heart.

Exercise is important too in the recovery period following a coronary. "Many physicians are now encouraging selected heart patients to engage in vigorous physical exercise once the damaged area of the heart has healed. This is a significant departure from the days when the emphasis in treatment was placed on sheltering the patient and protecting him from strenuous activity—which was regarded as absolutely dangerous."[1]

The most important thing for you to realize is that your efforts to prevent heart attacks must be done *now* to be most effective.

Your venous system also is given an assist by exercise. As your muscles contract they massage your veins and help the blood to flow uphill, against gravity, from your legs to your heart.

One final item on your heart and exercise—it has been rather well established that no amount of exercise, regardless of how strenuous, will injure a normal, healthy heart.

Exercise and Weight Control

Not many years ago, exercise was rejected as a means of controlling weight. Charts in textbooks illustrated how many mountains you had to

---

[1] Ralph Bugg, "They're Mending Hearts With Exercise," *Today's Health*, October, 1967, p. 50.

climb, how many hours of continuous woodchopping or how many hundred pushups were necessary to lose four or five pounds. We now recognize that it's not necessary to exercise to exhaustion and lose the weight all at once. You can attack the overweight problem in two ways. A pound of body fat is equal to about 3500 calories. (A calorie is a measure of energy. Food intake and energy expenditures are measured in calories.) During the period of one hour you can increase your caloric usage by approximately 100 calories by walking, as opposed to resting. By reducing your caloric intake by 100 calories a day at the same time, you can further your efforts to lose weight. This practice done daily will result in a loss of about 20 pounds in one year. Before going on any severe diet, however, consult your physician (Table 3).

Exercise and Menstruation

Misconceptions and superstitions have been associated with menstruation since earliest times. Primitive peoples though that if a menstruating woman touched a plant, the plant would die. In some tribes a woman was banned from her family's living quarters during the menstrual period, because an evil spirit was thought to possess her at this time. While these are obviously old wives' tales and not to be believed, there are many superstitions about menstruation that persist today. They are exemplified by statements such as: "Loss of menstrual blood weakens you." "Avoid exercise during menstruation." "Stay in bed at least one day." "Don't bathe or wash your hair and don't go swimming anytime during your period."

Here are some vital facts regarding exercise and menstruation:

1. It is important that you understand that menstrual cramps or dysmenorrhea are not normal. Mild cramps are often caused by factors *other* than menstruation itself. Poor posture is a factor, as is insufficient exercise. Poor posture, especially where hyperextension of the low back occurs, creates internal pressures. This can cause another problem—constipation.
2. Continue your exercises during menstruation because it increases circulation and aids in relieving the tension that helps to cause cramps.
3. Your mental attitude can cause your muscles to become tense and exaggerate the discomfort of cramps.
4. If you normally find cold water is a great shock to your system, you may wish to avoid swimming during your period. Many women, however, do swim throughout their period without ill effects.
5. Severe cramps require a physician's attention.

Miss Vera Milow, Director of Educational Services, Tampax, Inc., puts it this way in relating exercise to menstruation: "When your men-

EXERCISE AND SPECIAL HEALTH PROBLEMS   43

TABLE 3

Desirable Weights

Weight in Pounds According to Frame (In Indoor Clothing)

	HEIGHT (with shoes on) 1-inch heels Feet Inches	SMALL FRAME	MEDIUM FRAME	LARGE FRAME
Men of Ages 25 and Over	5 2	112–120	118–129	126–141
	5 3	115–123	121–133	129–144
	5 4	118–126	124–136	132–148
	5 5	121–129	127–139	135–152
	5 6	124–133	130–143	138–156
	5 7	128–137	134–147	142–161
	5 8	132–141	138–152	147–166
	5 9	136–145	142–156	151–170
	5 10	140–150	146–160	155–174
	5 11	144–154	150–165	159–179
	6 0	148–158	154–170	164–184
	6 1	152–162	158–175	168–189
	6 2	156–167	162–180	173–194
	6 3	160–171	167–185	178–199
	6 4	164–175	172–190	182–204
	HEIGHT (with shoes on) 2-inch heels Feet Inches	SMALL FRAME	MEDIUM FRAME	LARGE FRAME
Women of Ages 25 and Over	4 10	92– 98	96–107	104–119
	4 11	94–101	98–110	106–122
	5 0	96–104	101–113	109–125
	5 1	99–107	104–116	112–128
	5 2	102–110	107–119	115–131
	5 3	105–113	110–122	118–134
	5 4	108–116	113–126	121–138
	5 5	111–119	116–130	125–142
	5 6	114–123	120–135	129–146
	5 7	118–127	124–139	133–150
	5 8	122–131	128–143	137–154
	5 9	126–135	132–147	141–158
	5 10	130–140	136–151	145–163
	5 11	134–144	140–155	149–168
	6 0	138–148	144–159	153–173

For girls between 18 and 25, subtract 1 pound for each year under 25.

Courtesy of the Metropolitan Life Insurance Co.

1. The traditional 'military' posture has been "shoulder back, stomach in, etc.; what types of postural problems could an exaggeration of this position be likely to create?
2. Why are foot problems more common today than they were one hundred years ago?
3. How is the law of reciprocal innervation utilized in the dissipation of muscle cramps? What practical implications does this principle have for you?
4. Why does the text warn you to avoid certain exercises—particularly when football players use them in practice every day?

strual period comes, try to take it in stride without changing your daily activities of work and recreation. If you've been getting exercise regularly, even rather vigorous activity, there's no need to discontinue during this period. Common sense would also indicate that this is not the time to take up horseback riding for the first time, nor is it the best time to play field hockey for three hours when you've been playing just 30 minute stints."

Items for Discussion:
1. What is the relationship of exercise to posture?
2. What causes low back pain?
3. What's the role of exercise in:
   (a) foot problems
   (b) cardiovascular conditions
   (c) weight control
   (d) menstruation.

Selected Readings

Mix, Sheldon A. "Why Do We Torture Our Feet." *Today's Health*. May, 1964. p. 56.

Nolen, Jewell. "Problems of Menstruation." *Journal of Health, Physical Education, and Recreation*. Volume 36. October 1965. p. 65-66.

Phillips, Margery; Fox, Katherine; and Young C. "Sports Activity For Girls." *Journal of Health, Physical Education, and Recreation*. Volume 30. December 1959. p. 23-25.

"Sure You Can Lose Weight." *Changing Times*. May, 1966. p. 45.

Trulson, Martha F. and Stare, Frederick J. "The Great Balancing Act: Eating vs. Activity." *Today's Health*. June, 1963. p. 35.

CHAPTER 7

Rest or Sleep

Rest or sleep is a phenomenon which has puzzled man for centuries. Why do you sleep? Is it because night comes and with it, darkness? How much sleep do you need? Is sleep before midnight better than sleep after midnight? What part do dreams play in sleep?

Much research has been done on sleep but it is just recently that the instrumentation has become precise enough to develop valid data. While much remains to be learned, the findings are most interesting and have implications for your health.

Sleep is a restorative period which normally occurs once in a 24-hour period. It is through sleep that recovery of body tissues takes place, including the recovery from muscular fatigue due to activity.

While the obvious answer to the question, "Why do you sleep?" is, "Because I'm tired," it's not quite that simple. Man has within him a biological timeclock which triggers a myriad of chemical, physical and psychological changes. This cycle of sleep and wakefulness revolves around a period of about 24 hours. It is known as the circadian rhythm.

Although you may not sense the circadian rhythm in yourself, it is an important part of your life. It affects your efficiency as a student, your ability to concentrate, your judgment, and your reaction to stress. Jet travelers have experienced what it means to have this cycle disrupted. They may find themselves full of energy when they should be sleeping, or fatigued and irritable when they should be on their toes for the closing of a business deal. Anyone who was worked on a night shift in a factory can recall how difficult it was to become adjusted to the new regimen.

The circadian rhythm, while common to all people, is not exactly the same for each of you. Some individuals are most efficient early in the morning, while others can't really get under way until afternoon. You need to determine the most favorable times for you to do certain tasks. Just being aware of your own peaks and lows in performance is helpful in planning activities or in making adjustments to your mental and physical state of the moment.

Regarding the amount of sleep you need, it can be said that there are considerable individual differences. There's nothing magical about the number eight as in the statement, "You need eight hours of sleep for good health." Each person must determine his own sleep requirement. Some individuals operate efficiently with six or seven hours sleep while others require nine hours plus for best results.

Normal Sleep Patterns

Sleep patterns themselves are quite variable and yet have some fundamental components to what can be called "normal" sleep. The period just preceeding sleep is a drowsiness phase. It lasts about 20 minutes. Eyelids droop, yawning takes place and stretching is evident. This is followed by segments of deep sleep and dreaming. The dreaming is accompanied by rapid eye movements, and heightened secretions from various glands. Pulse and respiration increase and brain activity sometimes exceeds that of wakefulness. Despite the fact that the dream period is a stressful one, it is an important part of normal and restful sleep. It occupies about 20 per cent of the total sleep pattern and may occur anytime during the sleep period. The deep sleep portion usually occurs immediately following the period of drowsiness, but this varies from person to person. The fact that the deep sleep usually follows the period of drowsiness is the basis for the erroneus belief that sleep before midnight is better than sleep after midnight.

As college students it is important that you know this fact: reduced sleep is not a small reproduction of a full night's sleep. Your sleep pattern becomes disturbed when you reduce it markedly. This results in a less restful night and an accompanying lessened efficiency, when you awake.

The common practice of "pulling an all-nighter" to study for exams is a highly questionable practice. The resulting mental confusion from loss of sleep probably more than offsets, in a negative way, the increased amount of material you have studied for the test. Frequent use of the "all-nighters" can result in the beginnings of mental disturbances. In addition, the state of near-constant fatigue is a factor in lowered resistance to disease.

Fatigue

Symptoms of fatigue should not be ignored. Basically, there are two kinds of fatigue, acute and chronic. *Acute fatigue* is the result of physical activity. Normally, a college student recovers rather quickly from acute fatigue. If you enjoy a high level of fitness, recovery is a matter of minutes or a few hours. After a night's sleep you should enjoy complete recovery from acute fatigue.

Chronic fatigue is an other story. Chronic fatigue is your body's alarm system at work. When you feel tired most of the time and wake up after a night's rest still fagged out, something is wrong. It may be that you're developing what Dr. John S. Hopping, Medical Director at Wittenberg University, Springfield, Ohio, calls a "sleep deficit." When students consistently shortchange themselves, week after week and month after month, they're heading for trouble. As Dr. Hopping states, "Sleeping through a whole weekend or vacation period is not the solution. Getting a full night's rest of approximately eight hours for two weeks brings better results." A change of study habits to insure adequate sleep each 24-hour period is the next logical step.

Chronic fatigue also signals the onset of many diseases. Mononucleosis, the malady of college students across the nation, is directly related to chronic fatigue. Tuberculosis, infectious hepatitis, allergies, flu and pneumonia, head a long list of other conditions for which fatigue is symptomatic. Fatigue is prominent in cases of severe emotional disturbances too. So don't ignore chronic fatigue. Seek professional advice to determine its cause.

Drugs and Sleep

Since the beginnings of time man has related wakefulness to light, hope and pleasure; and sleep to darkness, loneliness and fear. Have you ever heard a modern mother say to her youngster, "Behave yourself or I'll send you to bed this minute"? Add this cultural legacy to the increased tensions of today's living and perhaps it's to be expected that we have sleep problems.

To increasing millions of Americans, including many college men and women, drugs are the answer to their quest for a "good night's sleep." Let's set the record straight. Sleeping pills do not induce normal sleep. According to Dr. Anthony Kales, Assistant Professor of Psychiatry, University of California at Los Angeles, certain sleeping pills depress dreaming sleep.[1] The use of the pills, furthermore, is habit forming. An imbalanced sleep pattern and fatigue are the result.

College students sometimes get involved with the use of sedatives by first taking amphetamines to stay awake to study. Often the student finds he cannot get to sleep after the study session. This is because of the disturbed sleep cycle caused by the stimulating effect of the amphetamine. He may try sleeping pills such as Sominex, Sleep-eze, or Nytol. These are mild and perfectly safe if used according to directions. But if they don't do the job, he may take drugs of a more potent type, such as barbiturates. When morning arrives he is groggy and so he takes an amphetamine such as dexedrine to get him going. Increased doses are needed as the individual develops a tolerance to the drugs. Before long the services of a psychiatrist will be needed to undo the damage.

Keep in mind that these college students and the many other adults who follow this procedure were not bent on self-destruction. They just sort of drifted into the situation, usually through a suggestion by a well-meaning friend. All of the drugs mentioned here have legitimate uses, when prescribed for individuals who have insomnia or tension problems. It is in their indiscriminate use that the dilemma arises.

---

[1]"Age, Health Affect Sleep Patterns," *Today's Health,* November, 1968, p. 77.

1. Students often sleep at highly irregular intervals; how does the circadian rhythm principle work against their overall effectiveness as students?
2. Which type of fatigue are students more prone to experience: chronic or acute? Which type, do you feel, has the greater detrimental effect over time?

Improve Your Sleep Patterns

These are suggested approaches to good sleep:
1. Try to cultivate a positive attitude toward sleep. Think of it as a pleasant, enjoyable portion of the 24-hour cycle in which your physical and mental powers are revitalized.
2. Establish a regular pattern of decreasing activity as the time for sleep approaches. A warm bath or reading a book may be part of the ritual. Avoid highly stimulating intellectual or physical activities just prior to retiring. Give yourself time to unwind.
3. Use your daily exercise period as a means of reducing nervous tension.
4. After you're in bed, reduce the tension in your muscles starting with your feet and preceeding to your head. (This will be explained in greater detail in Chapter 8.)
5. Don't panic when you feel you're about to have a poor night's sleep. A certain number of less restful nights are inevitable. Note the term "less restful." People who say they didn't sleep a wink all night are not making an accurate appraisal of their sleep patterns. Most of you sleep much more than you think, even on a poor night. The important thing is to not make a night of disturbed sleep worse by "pushing the panic button." If you're having difficulty in getting to sleep or wake up in the middle of the night wide-eyed and your mind aflood with thoughts, try a logical approach. Say to yourself, "So I'm not going to have a really great night's sleep. Why fret about it. Just calm down and try to relax." Think pleasant thoughts and refrain from dwelling on something that's bothering you. You'll soon drop off to sleep. Perhaps your sleep will continue through the night in a rather irregular pattern of sleep and wakefulness, but you'll not compound the problem by thrashing to and fro and worrying how you're going to carry on your daytime activities efficiently.

Selected Readings

Abarbanel, Albert. "What's in a Yawn?" *Today's Health*. May, 1964. p. 30.
"Age, Health Affect Sleep Patterns." *Today's Health*. November, 1968. p. 77.
Hicks, Clifford B. "Jet-Age Blues." *Today's Health*. November, 1966. p. 18.
Luce, Gay, Gaer and Segal, Julius. *Sleep*. New York: Coward McCann. 1966.
O'Brien, Robert. "Maybe You Need More Sleep." *Reader's Digest*. February, 1960. p. 102.

CHAPTER 8

Relaxation

"Jog a mile a day for your heart's sake." "Exercise and keep trim." "Get sufficient sleep and you'll revitalize yourself." These have been the prime messages directed at you up to this point. The benefits of exercise and restful sleep cannot be denied. But there are noteworthy benefits to be gained at another point on the continum—relaxation.

The vigorous activity of lifting barbells, performing a free exercise gymnastic routine or swimming a fifty-yard dash are examples of 100 per cent muscular stimulation. Sleep, at least deep sleep, represents the other end of the scale—zero activity in your muscles. Relaxation ranges from about 10 per cent to 0 per cent depending on your skill at doing it.

You may be saying, "But I relax too much now. That's why I'm gaining weight and need exercise, not more relaxation." You do need exercise, but you also need relaxation—*scientific relaxation*. Scientific relaxation is not playing golf or playing a game of cards or sitting under a shade tree on the campus. It's something quite different. Scientific relaxation is a method of eliminating tension from all the muscles of your body.

No one can learn much about scientific relaxation without coming across the name of Dr. Edmund Jacobson. Dr. Jacobson, a Chicago physician, first began research on relaxation in the early 1900's. He discovered that patients he was treating for nervous disorders exhibited a great deal of muscle tension at times when they were supposedly relaxed.[1]

Conversely, when Dr. Jacobson was able to teach these persons to reduce tension in specific muscle groups, the result was a reduction in general bodily nervousness. There were other benefits as well, including the easing of tension-caused headaches and the reduction in mental and physical fatigue.

Dr. Jacobson learned that the tension in muscles was the result of electrical energy in the form of nerve impulses coming from the muscles

---

[1] Edmund Jacobson, *You Must Relax*. New York: McGraw-Hill Book Co. 1962. p. 34.

and going to the central nervous system. Eventually he was able, through the cooperation of the Bell Telephone Laboratories, to devise an instrument which could accurately and objectively measure the tension in muscles. Thus, the basic understandings of scientific relaxation were formulated.

The physiological process which Dr. Jacobson came to understand is sometimes called the "fight or flight" mechanism. When primitive man saw a large beast approaching him he had to decide whether to attack or run away. In either case he needed to have all of his systems in a "go" condition. His muscles became tense and certain glands got him ready for action.

The same apparatus functions in modern man. When situations facing you are less than emergency in nature your muscles and glands react as in an emergency, but at a lower level. Even at these lower levels you develop much more muscle tension than you need.

The real problem, however, lies in that fact that the built-in stress of today's living causes you to over-react too often. Hardly a day passes that you are not subjected to tension-producing stimuli. An argument with a fellow-student, a letter from home, a disagreement with a professor, a television news program or a newspaper headline may cause you to clinch your teeth and tense your muscles. As the tension builds up in your muscles, a number of things occur. These include the throbbing headache, the nagging backache, difficulty in getting to sleep and that tired feeling—all the result of unneeded muscle tension.

In Dr. Jacobson's very readable book, "You Must Relax" first published in 1932 and revised in 1962, he describes how you can achieve relaxation. To profit from his lifetime of devotion to an amazing but simple principle, you must understand three terms:

1. *Progressive relaxation*. This is the process of attaining zero tension in the entire body by starting with one muscle group and proceeding muscle group by muscle group.
2. *Complete relaxation*. This is the end product of progressive relaxation.
3. *Differential relaxation*. This is the ability to relax unneeded muscle groups while other muscle groups are contracting.

Practicing Scientific Relaxation

Here's an example of how you can practice *progressive relaxation*. For best results you need an hour of time at mid-day or in late afternoon after classes. If you have a half hour or even fifteen minutes some progress can be made. Try to find a quiet place to do this. You will notice the word exercise was not added at the end of the last sentence. These are not exercises—but the reverse—no exercise whatsoever.

Sit in a chair—almost any kind will do. Allow yourself to slump down just a little, so your upper back is supported by the chair while the small of your back is away from the chairback slightly. Stop contracting your neck muscles and your head will fall forward, naturally. Rest your arms on the chair arms or on your thighs. Stretch your legs out in front of you and allow your toes to turn outward.

From this basic position you should begin to locate sites of tension in your muscles. With your palm down, bend either hand back toward your chest. Try to determine the area of tension. The strain at the wrist is not the tension point. It is farther up the forearm. Hold this position for three or four minutes until you can feel where the tension lies. Then, relax the hand and let it flop forward. Let go! Allow the tension to disappear. Maintain this new position for several minutes and then bend your hand back again and repeat the whole procedure. After doing this two or three times "let go" and then maintain a relaxed period for up to a half hour.

What you're doing through this process is learning where the tension is occurring and how to release the tension. To perfect the technique for just the muscles in one forearm may take you several days or several weeks. If you have an athletic background you will probably have better than average muscle awareness and progress fairly rapidly. Regardless of your aptitude, don't rush yourself and don't try to force yourself to relax. Just let it happen.

When you have been successful in relaxing the forearm, proceed to your biceps by flexing your arm at the elbow. You will no longer need to bend the hand but just "let go" right from the start. The leg muscles, seat muscles and abdominals can follow. Eventually you may even be able to relax your face and eye muscles. By this time you may develop the ability to blank your mind. Your *progressive relaxation* will be approaching *complete relaxation*. Complete relaxation, of course, can be only achieved by lying full length on your back. The best you can do in the chair is to develop *differential relaxation*. If you relaxed completely in the chair, you would slide to the floor.

Benefits of Relaxation

Just what's in it for you if after several weeks or months you gain some ability to achieve *complete relaxation?* Many benefits can be yours, according to Dr. Arthur H. Steinhaus, who has done recent research varifying Dr. Jacobson's original findings. Steinhaus, an eminent physiologist, for many years associated with George Williams College, Chicago, includes these outcomes of relaxation among his findings:[1]

(1) Reduction in insomnia
(2) Relief from nervous headaches
(3) Reduced sensation in pain and lessened reaction to loud sounds

---

[1] Arthur H. Steinhaus, "Facts and Theories of Neuromuscular Relaxation," *Quest,* December, 1964, p. 10.

(4) Diminution in habits such as smoking, nail biting and involuntary nervous muscle twitching or tics

(5) Ability to "blank" the mind at will and then return to difficult mental tasks with renewed vigor

Differential relaxation has many applications. The next time you drive your car, notice how much tension you have in your left leg and in other muscles which are not needed in driving. If you can learn to relax the unneeded muscles, you'll find yourself much more rested at the end of your trip.

Getting maximum power into your golf drives is accomplished by relaxing certain muscle groups while others contract. When your physical education instructor says, "You're too tight. Get some looseness in your swing," he's applying the principle of differential relaxation.

Yoga and Relaxation

While it is rather recently that physiologists have been able to explain the very complex interaction of muscle, nerve, central nervous system and glandular systems which operate in scientific relaxation, relaxation as an art has been practiced since prehistoric times. Yoga, which is of truly ancient origin, employs relaxation as a central theme for its followers. It is an amazing fact that without any of the precise electronic equipment available today, Yogic philosophers discovered the basic principles of relaxation. The method of reducing muscle tension using the Yogic approach is a little different from that used in scientific relaxation, but the results are quite similar.

Recall that with scientific relaxation you determined the locale of tension by tensing your muscles and then you "let go." No mental gymnastics or hypnotic suggestions were involved; in fact these were to be avoided according to Dr. Edmund Jacobson. The technique of Yoga is not quite the same.

Let's illustrate, using what Yogis call the Savasan or corpse pose (Figure 20). This is a backlying position with the body straight, arms extended near the body but not touching, and legs straight and apart about a foot. The feet are turned out slightly. You start relaxation of the entire body by *concentrating* first on your feet and toes. Concentration is the key. In a sense you're sending messages to your feet and toes telling them to lose their tension. Next you proceed to your leg muscles, on up to your arms and hands and continue upward to the trunk, the neck and face. Pay particular attention to your chin, cheeks, temples and finally the top of your head. Daily practice will enable you to gradually reduce the tension, literally from head to toe. In addition to assisting you to relax during the day, this technique is very helpful as a means of bridging the gap between wakefulness and deep sleep when you retire each night.

RELAXATION 53

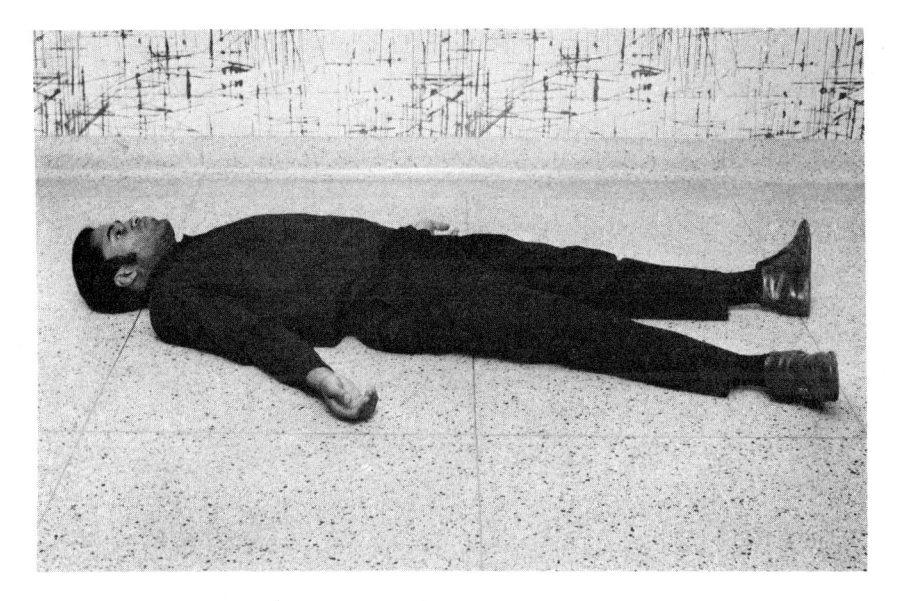

Figure 20. Yogic Corpse pose—Relaxation

From this same backlying position there is another Yogic practice which will help to reduce tension. Breathe slowly and rhythmically for a few moments and concentrate on your breathing. Your mind becomes detached from your previous thoughts and a calmness and serenity overcomes you. This is also helpful in gaining peaceful sleep.

There are many other aspects of Yoga which are gaining great appeal with people in the Western world. Much study, mediation and practice is necessary to reap the benefits of this age-old approach to life. In any event, you can now select from two methods of relaxation—scientific relaxation or relaxation through Yoga. In either case, let go!

As you complete the reading of this final chapter reflect a bit on some understandings you have gained. Hopefully these are some of the concepts or generalizations you have developed:

1. Exercise in some form has been a part of man's way of life since the beginning of time.
2. Your muscles respond favorably to exercise and waste away when not used.
3. Exercise can and should be enjoyable.
4. Different types of exercise bring varied results regarding strength, endurance and flexibility.
5. Care must be taken in selecting exercise equipment to most efficiently meet your exercise needs.

1. What danger is there in not being able to relax?
2. How is it realistically possible to relax under the pressures of a tight academic, athletic, and social schedule?
3. How can you apply the principle of differential relaxation to your daily routine?
4. Habits such as smoking, nail biting and involuntary nervous muscle twitching or tics seem to occur at some times more than others. How do they relate to the principles of relaxation discussed in this chapter?

6. Regular amounts of sleep based upon your individual requirements are important to good health.
7. Exercise is important in preventing health problems related to posture, foot maladies, heart disease and menstrual difficulties.
8. While exercise is important to your health, the ability to relax is equally valuable.

One final suggestion—start now to make exercise a regular part of your weekly, if not daily, routine. An increased zest for living will be your invaluable reward.

ITEMS FOR DISCUSSION:
1. What is scientific relaxation?
2. What are some benefits of relaxation?
3. How does Yoga contribute to relaxation?

SELECTED READINGS
ALDIN. *Yoga For Perfect Health.* New York: Pyramid Books. 1957.
JACOBSON, EDMUND. *You Must Relax.* New York: McGraw-Hill Book Company. 1962.
VISHNUDEVANANDA, SWAMI. *The Complete Book of Yoga.* New York: Bell Publishing Co. Inc. 1960.
YESUDIAN, SELVARAJAN and HAICH, ELIZABETH. *Yoga and Health.* New York: Harper and Row. 1953.

Index

Abdominal muscles:
  isometrics, 38
Aerobics:
  cycling, 15
  definition, 11, 14
  running, 14, 15
  training effect, 14
American Medical Association:
  fitness and longevity, 22
  hot weather exercise hints, 31
Atrophy:
  definition, 7

Blood clot:
  see embolus, 41
Body mechanics:
  definition, 39

Calisthenics:
  flexibility, 14
  general endurance, 14
  local endurance, 14
  training effect, 14
Calorie:
  definition, 42
Calories:
  exercise, 42
Capillarization:
  definition, 41
Cardiovascular systems:
  endurance, 9
Cardiovascular test:
  procedure for, 28
Circadian rhythm:
  sleep, 45
Coronary heart attack:
  cause, 41

Deep knee bends:
  ill effects from, 40
Drugs:
  sleep, 47

Electrocardiograph test:
  physical examination, 27
Embolus:
  definition, 41
Endurance:
  definition, 9
  development of, 11

  general, 9
  local, 9
Exercise:
  benefits, 18, 19
  cardiovascular and respiratory
    changes due to, 9, 10
  colonial America, 5
  coronary heart attack, 41
  enjoyment, 4
  fatigue, 10, 19
  Greeks, 4, 5
  health, 4
  heat exhaustion, dehydration, 31
  history of, 4
  hot weather hints, 31
  longevity, 22
  measuring effects of, 28
  menstruation, 42
  mental tension, 19
  military preparedness, 5
  motivation for, 4
  oxygen debt, 10
  physical development, 5
  professional strong men, 5
  quality of living, 22
  second-wind phenomenon, 10
  social values, 5
  Socrates, 5
  through sports participation, 16
  types of, 10
  weight control, 41
Exercises:
  ones to avoid, 40
  selection of, 23, 24, 25, 26
Exercise and posture:
  low back pain, 37
  round shoulders, 36
Exercise equipment:
  consumer guides, 32
  electronic gadgets, 32
  exercise bicycles, 30, 31
  Exergene, 30
  isometrics, 32
  isotonics, 32
  sweat clothing, 31
Exercise programs:
  evaluation of, 26

INDEX

Fatigue:
　acute, 46
　chronic, 46, 47
Flexibility:
　back muscles, 38
　benefits, 19
　example of, 19
　programs for college women, 20
Flexibility exercises:
　injury prevention, 40
Foot health:
　tips for, 39
Foot problems:
　flexibility, 39

Health Clubs:
　types, 33
Health Spas:
　benefits, 34, 35
　equipment, 33
　sauna bath, 35
　Turkish steam room, 35
Heart Attacks:
　recovery and exercise, 41
Heart rate:
　average for men, 28
　average for women, 28
Hypertrophy:
　definition, 18

Isometrics:
　definition, 10
　general endurance, 11
　local endurance, 11
　sports, 26
　strength,
Isotonics:
　definition, 11
　flexibility, 11
　overload principle, 11

Jogging:
　benefits, 24
Judo:
　college men, 1
　college women, 4

Karate:
　college men, 1
　college women, 4
Kraus-Weber tests:
　flexibility, 19

Law of reciprocal innervation:
　explanation, 40
Low back pain:
　cause, 37, 38
　hyperextension of lumbar spine, 38
　Yoga exercise, 39

Menstruation
　exercise, 42
Muscles:
　atrophy, 7
　elasticity, flexibility, 7
　lengthening contraction, 7, 8
　overload principle, 9
　shortening contraction, 7, 8
　tone, tonus, 7
　warmup, 40
Orthopedist:
　foot problems, 39
Overload principle:
　definition, 9

Physical examination:
　exercise programs, 27
Physical fitness:
　Civil War, 5
　definition, 18
　draft rejections, 5
　World War I, 5
　World War II, 5
Physical training:
　Swedish and German gymnastics, 5
Posture:
　abdominal muscles, 38
President's Council on Physical Fitness:
　exercises, 14

Relaxation:
　benefits, 51, 52
　complete, 50
　differential, 50
　muscle tension, 50
　practice of, 50, 51
　progressive, 50
　scientific, 49
　Yoga, 52, 53
Respiratory system:
　endurance, 9
Royal Canadian Air Force Physical
　　Fitness:
　exercises, 14
Running:
　benefits, 24

Scientific relaxation:
　definition, 49
Sleep:
　dreaming, 46
　drugs, 47
　effect on studying, 46
　normal, 46
　rapid eye movements, 46
　types, 45, 46
Sleep patterns:
　ways to improve, 48

INDEX

Sports, games:
    tension reduction, 25
    values, 25
Strength:
    definition, 9
    development of, 11
Stretching exercises:
    pain reduction, 40
Swimming:
    common cold, 25
    sedative effects, 25
    strength endurance, 25
    training effect, 25

Walking:
    benefits, 24, 25
Warmup:
    methods, 40
Weight:
    desirable levels for men, 43
    desirable levels for women, 43

Weight lifting:
    definition, 16
Weight reduction:
    massage machine, 51
    sweat clothing, 31
Weight training:
    benefits, 26
    definition, 16
    flexibility, 16
    general endurance, 16
    local endurance, 16
    overload principle, 26

Yoga:
    participation by college women, 4
    relaxation, 52, 53
    tension reduction, 52
Yoga exercise:
    low back pain, 39